Hallux Rigidus

Editor

ERIC GIZA

FOOT AND ANKLE CLINICS

www.foot.theclinics.com

Consulting Editor
MARK S. MYERSON

September 2015 • Volume 20 • Number 3

ELSEVIER

1600 John F. Kennedy Boulevard • Suite 1800 • Philadelphia, Pennsylvania, 19103-2899

http://www.theclinics.com

FOOT AND ANKLE CLINICS Volume 20, Number 3
September 2015 ISSN 1083-7515, ISBN-13: 978-0-323-39563-2

Editor: Jennifer Flynn-Briggs
Developmental Editor: Meredith Clinton

Foot and Ankle Clinics (ISSN 1083-7515) is published quarterly by Elsevier, Inc., 360 Park Avenue South, New York, NY 10010-1710. Months of issue are March, June, September, and December. Periodicals postage paid at New York, NY, and additional mailing offices. Subscription price per year is $315.00 (US individuals), $421.00 (US institutions), $155.00 (US students), $360.00 (Canadian individuals), $506.00 (Canadian institutions), $215.00 (Canadian students), $460.00 (international individuals), $506.00 (international institutions), and $215.00 (international students). To receive student/resident rate, orders must be accompanied by name of affiliated institution, date of term, and the *signature* of program/residency coordinator on institution letterhead. Orders will be billed at individual rate until proof of status is received. Foreign air speed delivery is included in all *Clinics* subscription prices. All prices are subject to change without notice. **POSTMASTER:** Send address changes to *Foot and Ankle Clinics*, Elsevier Health Sciences Division, Subscription Customer Service, 3251 Riverport Lane, Maryland Heights, MO 63043. **Customer Service: 1-800-654-2452 (US and Canada). From outside of the United States and Canada, call 314-447-8871. Fax: 314-447-8029. E-mail: JournalsCustomerService-usa@ elsevier.com (for print support); JournalsOnlineSupport-usa@elsevier.com (for online support).**

Reprints. For copies of 100 or more, of articles in this publication, please contact the Commercial Reprints Department, Elsevier Inc., 360 Park Avenue South, New York, NY 10010-1710. Tel.: 212-633-3874; Fax: 212-633-3820; E-mail: reprints@elsevier.com.

Contributors

CONSULTING EDITOR

MARK S. MYERSON, MD
Director, The Institute for Foot and Ankle Reconstruction, Mercy Medical Center, Baltimore, Maryland

EDITOR

ERIC GIZA, MD
Chief, Foot and Ankle Surgery; Associate Professor of Orthopaedic Surgery, Department of Orthopaedics, University of California, Davis, Sacramento, California

AUTHORS

BOLESLAW CZACHOR, MD
Fellow, Department of Foot and Ankle Surgery, Thomas Jefferson University, The Rothman Institute for Orthopaedics, Philadelphia, Pennsylvania

CONNOR DELMAN, BS
Department of Orthopaedics, University of California, Davis, Sacramento, California

J. KENT ELLINGTON, MD, MS
OrthoCarolina, Foot and Ankle Institute, Charlotte, North Carolina

CHAD M. FERGUSON, MD
Department of Orthopaedic Surgery, Carolinas Medical Center, Charlotte, North Carolina

ERIC GIZA, MD
Chief, Foot and Ankle Surgery; Associate Professor of Orthopaedic Surgery, Department of Orthopaedics, University of California, Davis, Sacramento, California

KAMRAN S. HAMID, MD, MPH
Chief Resident, Department of Orthopaedic Surgery, Wake Forest School of Medicine, Winston-Salem, North Carolina

THOMAS HARRIS, MD
Congress Medical Associates, Foot and Ankle Surgery, Harbor-UCLA, Pasadena; Department of Orthopaedics, Harbor-UCLA, Torrance, California

CARL T. HASSELMAN, MD
Clinical Assistant Professor, University of Pittsburgh Medical Center, Three Rivers Orthopaedic Associates, Pittsburgh, Pennsylvania

KENNETH J. HUNT, MD
Assistant Professor, Department of Orthopedics, Stanford University School of Medicine, Redwood City, California

ALEX J. KLINE, MD
Clinical Assistant Professor, University of Pittsburgh Medical Center, Three Rivers
Orthopaedic Associates, Pittsburgh, Pennsylvania

CHRIS KREULEN, MD
Assistant Professor of Orthopaedic Surgery, Department of Orthopaedics, University of
California, Davis, Sacramento, California

REMESH KUNNASEGARAN, MBChB (Glasgow), MRCS (Glasgow)
Department of Orthopaedics, Tan Tock Seng Hospital, Singapore, Singapore

DOUGLAS E. LUCAS, DO
Clinical Instructor, Department of Orthopedics, Stanford University School of Medicine,
Redwood City, California

THOMAS MITTLMEIER, MD, PhD
Professor, Department of Trauma and Reconstructive Surgery; Director, Center of
Surgery, University Hospital Rostock, Rostock, Germany

MARK S. MYERSON, MD
Director, The Institute for Foot and Ankle Reconstruction, Mercy Medical Center,
Baltimore, Maryland

INES PANZNER, MD
Foot and Ankle Section, University Center of Orthopaedics and Traumatology, University
Hospital Carl Gustav Carus Dresden, Dresden, Germany

SELENE G. PAREKH, MD, MBA
Associate Professor, Department of Orthopaedic Surgery, North Carolina Orthopaedic
Clinic, Duke University School of Medicine, Durham, North Carolina

ANTHONY PERERA, MBChB, FRCS (Orth)
Foot and Ankle Surgeon, Foot and Ankle Clinic, Spire Cardiff Hospital, Cardiff, United
Kingdom

STEVEN M. RAIKIN, MD
Director and Attending Orthopaedic Surgeon, Department of Foot and Ankle Surgery;
Director, Foot and Ankle Service; Professor, Orthopaedic Surgery, Thomas Jefferson
University, The Rothman Institute for Orthopaedics, Philadelphia, Pennsylvania

STEFAN RAMMELT, MD, PhD
Professor, Head of Foot and Ankle Section, University Center of Orthopaedics and
Traumatology, University Hospital Carl Gustav Carus Dresden, Dresden, Germany

TIMO SCHMID, MD
Fellow, University of British Columbia, Vancouver, British Columbia, Canada

RAHEEL SHARIFF, FRCS (Tr & Orth)
Consultant Orthopaedic Surgeon, Trauma and Orthopaedic Surgery, Central Manchester
University Hospitals NHS Foundation Trust, Manchester, United Kingdom

MARTIN SULLIVAN, MD, FRACS
Fellowship Director, Foot and Ankle Clinic, St. Vincents Clinic, Darlinghurst, Sydney,
Australia

GOWREESON THEVENDRAN, MBChB (Bristol), MFSEM (UK), FRCS Ed (Tr & Orth)
Department of Orthopaedics, Tan Tock Seng Hospital, Singapore, Singapore

RICHARD WALTER, FRCS (Orth)
Foot and Ankle Fellow, North Bristol NHS Trust, Bristol, United Kingdom

TIBOR WARGANICH, MD
Resident, Department of Orthopaedics, Harbor-UCLA, Torrance, California

BRIAN S. WINTERS, MD
Attending Orthopaedic Surgeon, Rothman Institute for Orthopaedics, Egg Harbor
Township, New Jersey

ALASTAIR YOUNGER, MD, FRCSC
Professor, Department of Orthopaedics, University of British Columbia, Vancouver,
British Columbia, Canada

Contents

 This article contains videos on intraoperative demonstration

Hallux rigidus is a painful condition of the great toe characterized by re-striction of the metatarsophalangeal joint arc of motion and progressive osteophyte formation. Precise cause of hallux rigidus remains under debate. Anatomic variations and historical, clinical, and radiographic find-ings have been implicated in the development and progression of hallux rigidus. Radiologic findings associated with hallux rigidus include meta-tarsal head osteochondral defects, altered metatarsal head morphology, and an elevated hallux interphalangeus angle measure. Associated histor-ical findings include a positive family history and history of trauma to the joint. An understanding of relevant anatomy and pathophysiology is essen-tial during the approach to hallux rigidus treatment.

Hallux rigidus is the most commonly occurring arthritic condition of the foot and is marked by pain, limited motion in the sagittal plane of the first metatarsophalangeal joint and varying degrees of functional impairment. In conjunction with clinical findings, radiographic grading helps guide ther-apeutic choices. Nonsurgical management with anti-inflammatory medi-cations, corticosteroid injections, or shoewear and activity modifications can be successful in appropriately selected patients. Patients with more severe disease or refractory to conservative management may benefit from surgical intervention. Operative options range from joint-preserving procedures (eg, cheilectomy with or without associated osteotomies) to joint-altering procedures (eg, arthroplasty or arthrodesis).

Hallux rigidus, the most common degenerative disorder of the foot, is accountable for abnormality of gait and restriction of activity levels and daily function. This article describes and reviews the available literature on nonoperative modalities available in the treatment of hallux rigidus, including manipulation and intra-articular injections, shoe modifications and orthotics, physical therapy, and experimental therapies.

Associated deformities are corrected and greater defects are filled with interposition autograft or allograft. Fusion is generally obtained with screws, staples, and/or low-profile plates. Complications include infection, osteonecrosis, implant protrusion or failure, nonunion, and malunion, the latter two each occurring in approximately 6% of cases. The medium-term results of first MTP joint fusion indicate mostly good functional results with success rates of approximately 90%.

First metatarsophalangeal joint disorder is a common cause of chronic forefoot pain that is frequently encountered in the orthopedic clinic. Numerous surgical techniques have been described to improve patient pain and function in this regard, including prosthetic joint replacement, resection arthroplasty, and arthrodesis. When these procedures fail, surgeons can be confronted with significant first metatarsal bone loss/defects. First metatarsophalangeal joint fusion remains the gold standard and, in the setting of significant bone loss, the use of structural bone graft must be considered in order to restore length to the first ray and the normal biomechanics of the foot.

Metatarsus elevatus and gastrocnemius tightness contribute to the development of functional hallux rigidus. Although several osteotomies have been described for functional hallux rigidus, certain osteotomies are commonly used in practice for the correction of functional hallux rigidus, a long first metatarsal or an elevated metatarsal, or an unstable tarsometatarsal joint. Proximal plantarflexion osteotomy is used only in the presence of an elevated first metatarsal with a limit to dorsiflexion but without the presence of arthritis at the first metatarsophalangeal joint. In the presence of arthritis at the metatarsophalangeal joint, the decision is between an oblique distal metatarsal osteotomy and the shortening periarticular osteotomy.

Multiple treatment options exist for the management of late-stage hallux rigidus. The goals of treatment are pain reduction and restoration of function. Arthrodesis remains the treatment of choice, but recent advances support the use of first metatarsophalangeal hemiarthroplasty as a viable and successful option in properly selected patients in whom preservation of motion and function are desirable.

Hallux rigidus is the most common arthritic malady to afflict the foot. A host of nonoperative measures can alleviate pain, and with failure of conservative treatment, joint preserving and joint sacrificing procedures can be used to treat signs and symptoms. Although arthrodesis is an effective pain-relieving operation, loss of motion at the hallux metatarsophalangeal joint may limit the patient's function and can be an unacceptable solution. Interposition arthroplasty, as described originally as the modified Keller procedure, or including one of a host of varieties, can offer a motion-preserving alternative to arthrodesis.

FOOT AND ANKLE CLINICS

RELATED INTEREST

Orthopedic Clinics of North America
July 2015 (Vol. 46, No. 3)
Asif M. Ilyas, Saqib Rehman, Giles R. Scuderi and
Felasfa M. Wodajo, *Editors*

THE CLINICS ARE NOW AVAILABLE ONLINE!
Access your subscription at:
www.theclinics.com

Preface

Hallux Rigidus

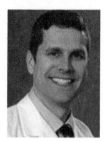

Eric Giza, MD
Editor

During my first rotation as a PGY-2 resident in the late 1990s, I specifically remember being told by a (now retired) faculty, "The only thing that you can do with hallux rigidus is fuse it, or cut the bump off!" Certainly, first MTP fusion and cheilectomy are still effective procedures for the properly selected patient. Fortunately though, for many halluces in this world, there have been significant advancements in the treatment of foot and ankle maladies over the past twenty years. The complexity of the treatment of hallux rigidus has improved not only with the myriad of surgical interventions, but also with an increased understanding of the pathology of the disorder on the molecular, anatomic, and biomechanical levels.

The readers of this issue of *Foot and Ankle Clinics of North America* will find a comprehensive review of the current treatment options for hallux rigidus that have been authored by surgeons with a vast experience and knowledge of the condition. The variety of approaches by the different authors demonstrates that hallux rigidus is not just a simple arthritic condition, but it reflects the modern cultural desire of our patients, who would like to maintain mobility and function over the course of their lifetime. Along with fusion and salvage techniques, the reader will find some compelling articles about joint-preserving techniques.

I would like to thank Dr Myerson for honoring me with the duty of editing this issue, and I also thank our authors for their time and contributions. Mark Twain once wrote, "Whenever you find yourself on the side of the majority, it is time to pause and reflect."

Foot Ankle Clin N Am 20 (2015) xiii–xiv
http://dx.doi.org/10.1016/j.fcl.2015.07.001
1083-7515/15/$ – see front matter © 2015 Published by Elsevier Inc.

foot.theclinics.com

I am delighted to be part of our foot and ankle community that has not just followed the former "majority" and has transcended beyond "just fusing or cutting the bump off."

Eric Giza, MD
Foot and Ankle Surgery
University of California, Davis
Department of Orthopaedics
4860 Y Street, Suite 3800
Sacramento, CA 95817, USA

E-mail address:
egiza@ucdavis.edu

Hallux Rigidus
Relevant Anatomy and Pathophysiology

Douglas E. Lucas, DO, Kenneth J. Hunt, MD*

KEYWORDS

- Metatarsal head • Metatarsus primus elevatus • Arthritis • Great toe • Bunion
- Hallux valgus • Forefoot pain • Osteochondral defect

KEY POINTS

- Hallux rigidus is a common, painful condition characterized by restricted range of motion and progressive osteophyte formation.
- Family history of hallux rigidus increases the likelihood of having bilateral disease.
- Trauma or multiple episodes of microtrauma seem to play a role in the development of most cases of hallux rigidus.
- Radiographic factors found to have an association with hallux rigidus include evidence of osteochondritis dessicans, flattened or chevron-shaped metatarsal head, and an elevated hallux interphalangeus angle.

 This article contains videos on intraoperative demonstration at http://www. foot.theclinics.com/

INTRODUCTION

Hallux rigidus is a painful, degenerative condition of the metatarsophalangeal (MTP) joint of the great toe that is characterized by restricted range of motion and progressive osteophyte formation.[1–7] Hallux rigidus was first described by Davies-Colley in 1887 as hallux flexus and Cotterill first coined the condition as hallux rigidus shortly afterward in 1888.[8,9] Since that time, several anatomic, historical, and radiologic findings have been investigated as etiologic factors.[10] Although trauma is a commonly accepted cause for a monoarthritis, other pathophysiologic features of hallux rigidus have evidence supporting their role in the disorder, its development, and its progression. As newer treatment techniques and implants emerge for the treatment of hallux rigidus, outcomes will be optimized if the treating physician is equipped with a

The authors have nothing to disclose.
Department of Orthopedics, Stanford University School of Medicine, 450 Broadway Street, Redwood City, CA 94063, USA
* Corresponding author. 450 Broadway Street, MC 6342, Redwood City, CA 94063.
E-mail address: kjhunt@stanford.edu

comprehensive understanding of the relevant anatomy, pathophysiology, and patient risk factors contributing to symptomatic hallux rigidus.

ANATOMY AND KINEMATICS OF THE HALLUX METATARSOPHALANGEAL JOINT COMPLEX

The anatomy of the first metatarsal is unique and its shape may play a significant role in the development of hallux rigidus.[10,11] The first metatarsal head is a large transversely flattened quadrilateral structure with dorsoplantar diameter smaller than transverse.[12] This is unique to the first metatarsal because the lesser metatarsal heads are longer in the dorsoplantar direction and smaller in the transverse plane. The articular surface is continuous but functionally divided into superior and inferior fields (**Fig. 1**A). The superior field is a convex dome larger than its phalangeal counterpart. Dorsally the dome rises above the level of the metatarsal shaft and ends in a smooth border. The inferior field is larger than the superior. It is divided into two sloped articulations for the sesamoids by an anterior to posteriorly directed ridge. The ridge or cristae is generally located at the junction of the lateral one-third and medial two-thirds of the articular surface. The uneven distribution of surface area makes room for the larger tibial sesamoid with a more pronounced groove in the metatarsal head.

The proximal phalanx of the great toe articulates with the first metatarsal head. It has a large concave articular surface that is directed more transversely to match the head of the first metatarsal. Tubercles exist just off the articular surface for insertions of tendons from the following muscles: extensor hallucis brevis, intrinsics muscles of the foot, flexor hallucis brevis, adductor halluces, and abductor halluces.

The sesamoids plantar to the first metatarsal head are constant. There are two sesamoids located within the plantar plate capsuloligamentous complex. The medial or tibial sesamoid is generally larger and more ovoid in shape, whereas the lateral or fibular is smaller, more round, and located more proximally.[13] The nonarticular surface serves as an important insertion point for multiple structures. The articular surface does so with the corresponding sloped articulations of the metatarsal head.

The plantar plate of the first MTP joint is a critical structure of the capsuloligamentous complex that provides stability to the hallux. It serves as an attachment for ligaments and tendons medially and laterally and when disrupted can have devastating effects on joint stability and function. The position of the structure is consistent and well described with static insertion averaging 0.3-mm distal to the joint line into the proximal phalanx and 1.73-mm proximal to the joint line into the metatarsal head.[13]

When examined together the surfaces making up the MTP joint demonstrate unique relationships. Shereff and colleagues[14] cadaveric work on first MTP joint

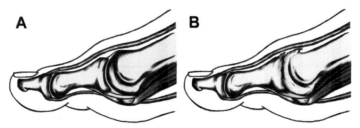

Fig. 1. (*A*) Drawing of normal anatomy at the hallux metatarsophalangeal joint. (*B*) Drawing of joint with advanced hallux rigidus demonstrating dorsal osteophyte, narrowing of the joint space, and subcortical irregularities. (*Courtesy of* Nathan T. Formaini, DO, Holy Cross Orthopedic Institute, Fort Lauderdale, FL.)

kinematics demonstrated the impressive motion available to this joint. The control group had a mean sagittal plane arc of 111° and 76° of dorsiflexion with transvers plane translation equal to 15% of the width of the metatarsal head. This range of motion demands that the static and dynamic restraints of the joint carefully balance motion and stability. The hallux rigidus group within this study demonstrated significantly less motion with a mean sagittal arc of 69°, dorsiflexion of 49°, and transverse translation less than half that of the control group. The authors concluded that the scarring of the joint capsule and abnormal centers of rotation resulted in abnormal compression forces across the joint and decreased range of motion.[14] These forces lead to the clinical and radiographic findings often found in patients with hallux rigidus.

CLINICAL FEATURES OF HALLUX RIGIDUS

Patients with hallux rigidus present in a predictable manner. The universal finding is the presence of a dorsal osteophyte on the first metatarsal (see **Fig. 1**B; **Fig. 2**, Video 1). Clinical presentation can vary, but the common clinical signs and symptoms are well described in the literature.[2,10,15,16]

- Pain is frequently the presenting symptom and begins with pain only at extremes of motion but as the condition progresses eventually midrange of motion becomes painful.[2]
- Restricted MTP motion is a hallmark clinical finding with dorsiflexion affected earlier and to a greater extent. The goal of surgical treatment is to restore the sagittal arc of motion (Video 2)
- A painful dorsal prominence is frequently noticed and can be troublesome with shoe wear. Functional deficits are noticed early as range of motion decreases.
- Inability to dorsiflex the great toe results in a decreased ability to rise onto the toes, roll through the forefoot, or run.

CLINICAL ETIOLOGIC FACTORS

There is inconsistency in the literature regarding the pertinent clinical and associated radiographic features, demographics, cause, and clinical findings of hallux rigidus.[5,10] Herein, we describe the anatomic features of hallux rigidus, including those postulated, and often supported, as causative factors. The true cause is not universally agreed on and numerous etiologic factors have been discussed in the literature with little objective evidence to qualify most of them.[1]

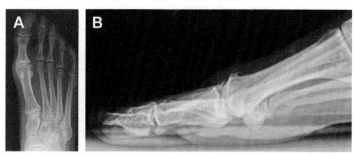

Fig. 2. Standing (A) anteroposterior and (B) lateral radiographs of a patient with hallux rigidus.

Trauma

A memorable traumatic event, such as an intra-articular fracture or a series of minor events (ie, stubbed toes), has been suggested as the most common cause of hallux rigidus.[1,3–5] Despite the suggested correlation, historical studies only indicate a 12% to 14% incidence of recalled trauma in hallux rigidus cohorts.[17] Because of the duration of the disease and methodology of many studies, recall bias likely contributes to falsely low numbers.

Jack[18] was first to describe the concept of multiple microtraumas as a cause for hallux rigidus. Although a single traumatic event may be memorable, multiple microtraumas may not be. The adult population is not only more likely to have suffered multiple microtraumas over time but is also more likely to suffer recall bias in questionnaires. Both of these reasons make trauma less likely to be identified in adults, but this does not seem to be the case for adolescents.

Coughlin and Shurnas[10] found in their study on etiology that adolescent patients with unilateral disease are likely to have reported acute trauma. They also found in the same study that if trauma was reported, the disease was unilateral in 78% of patients regardless of age. Thus, in unilateral cases, either a single macrotraumatic event or multiple microevents is likely to play a role in the development of hallux rigidus.

First Ray Hypermobility

First ray hypermobility was also suggested as a cause by Jack.[18] The original article, however, provided no method to objectively define the measurement or clinically evaluate the condition. Klaue and colleagues[19] were the first to describe a classification system using objective measurements. Coughlin and Shurnas[20] used a similar method to measure hypermobility and found none in a small cohort of seven patients with hallux rigidus.

Metatarsus Primus Elevatus

An elevated first ray was suggested by Lambrinudi[21] in 1938 as associated with hallux rigidus based on a single case report. This condition is defined as elevation of the first ray on the lateral standing radiograph when compared with the position of the second metatarsal. Historically considered a primary pathology in association with hallux rigidus, recommended surgical options frequently included a first metatarsal osteotomy to correct the deformity.[15,17,22]

Meyer and coworkers[23] and Horton and coworkers[3] independently found that metatarsus primus elevatus (MPE) is a normal finding and is present no more frequently in patients with hallux rigidus than in a control group.

More recent opinions view medial column elevation as consequence of limited dorsiflexion of the great toe MTP joint.[1–3,10,20] As a sequelae of disease progression MPE can be seen in grades 3 and 4 radiographs more frequently than in control subjects.[10]

Coughlin and Horton both noted that if elevatus was present preoperatively it improved significantly after hallux rigidus correction procedures without metatarsal osteotomy.[2,3,20] Hunt and Anderson[24] showed a similar correction in MPE after cheilectomy combined with phalanx osteotomy.

Family History

A positive family history likely plays a role in the development of hallux rigidus. Although recall bias is certain to limit data accuracy in retrospective studies, some conclusions can be drawn with available data. The series by Coughlin and Shurnas[10] demonstrates that a positive family history was reported 67% of the time and those with a positive family history had bilateral symptoms 95% of the time. They also concluded that family history does not seem to affect age of onset.[10]

Equinus and Pes Planus

A tight heel cord and pes planus were both identified as potential etiologies for hallux rigidus in early literature.[15,25,26] Coughlin and Shurnas[20] noted in a series that used clinical examination and a Harris Mat evaluation that pes planus was not found to be more common in those with hallux rigidus when compared with historical averages from Harris and Beath.[27] A second study by the same authors looked at 110 patients treated for hallux rigidus. They found only four with less than 5° of dorsiflexion with the knee extended and performed no lengthening. They concluded that equinus was not more common in their cohort than published rates of equinus in the general public.[10,28]

Hallux Valgus

Hallux valgus has been identified in conjunction with hallux rigidus 12% of the time in the series by Coughlin and Shurnas.[10] Although not frequent enough to be considered an etiologic factor for hallux rigidus, it should be considered as an associated variable. When the two present together surgical treatment has been described to address both deformities simultaneously.[24]

Hallux Valgus Interphalangeus

An elevated hallux valgus interphalangeus angle has been evaluated as an associated radiographic and clinical finding of hallux rigidus.[24] This association was seen 90% of the time in the series by Coughlin and Shurnas.[10] They suggested that as the first metacarpophalangeal joint becomes more resistant to transverse plane motion increased stresses through the interphalangeal joint lead to an elevated measurement. This reinforces the historic findings of a hypermobile interphalangeal joint in adolescent patients that becomes deformed and degenerative over time as the increased transverse plane stress takes a toll on the joint.[25] Phalangeal osteotomies have been described that take this deformity into account when treating early rigidus from the distal aspect of the joint.[24]

COMMON ASSOCIATED RADIOGRAPHIC FINDINGS

After physical examination, the most frequently implemented objective assessment of hallux rigidus includes radiographs. It is common to obtain several radiographic views of the hallux MTP joint with weight-bearing radiographs (anteroposterior; lateral; oblique; and, when indicated, sesamoid views). Hallux rigidus is most often characterized by dorsal osteophytes of both the metatarsal head and the base of the proximal phalanx as seen in **Figs. 2** and **3**. Several other radiographic features have also been found to be associated with hallux rigidus.

Flat or Chevron-Shaped Metatarsal Head

Nonspherical hallux morphology has been shown to be associated with hallux rigidus.[1,4] Although the natural incidence of different morphologies is unknown, Coughlin and Shurnas[10] demonstrated a seemingly high (74%) incidence of flattened, squared, or chevron-shaped metatarsal heads in a cohort of patients with hallux rigidus. Additionally, a radiographic study on cadaveric specimens with and without hallux rigidus demonstrated that metatarsal heads with a larger radius of curvature (flatter than normal) were found in specimens with hallux rigidus.[29] Most recently

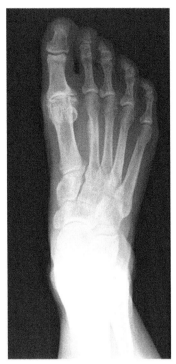

Fig. 3. Standing anteroposterior radiograph demonstrates periarticular osteophyte formation.

Hunt and Anderson[24] evaluated head morphology in their series looking at biplanar phalanx osteotomies for hallux rigidus and noted that patients had a flat or chevron-shaped metatarsal shape 79% of the time, which supports Coughlin's previous findings.

Metatarsal Osteochondritis Dessicans

Osteochondritis dessicans (OCD) of the metatarsal head continues to be investigated in hallux rigidus literature. Despite its unclear cause, OCD is frequently found on imaging when evaluating hallux rigidus.[1,3,5,11,16,22] McMaster[5] demonstrated that 100% of a young cohort averaging 21 years of age showed radiographic evidence of OCD and concluded that a single episode of macrotrauma or multiple microtraumas were responsible for 100% of the hallux rigidus in his series. Goodfellow[16] described the transition from OCD to hallux rigidus, postulating that bone remodeling during the healing of an OCD results in the chevron or flattened metatarsal head. Metatarsal OCD can be seen on radiographs, MRI, and during arthroscopy as seen in **Figs. 4** and **5**.

Metatarsal Length

An excessively long or short metatarsal was thought to put extra stress on the MTP joint and was implicated in the development of hallux rigidus in early literature.[9,23,26] An MRI study on cadaveric specimens with hallux rigidus in 1999 refuted this finding.[11]

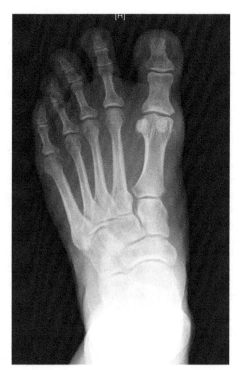

Fig. 4. Standing anteroposterior radiograph demonstrating osteochondritis dessicans in the metatarsal head.

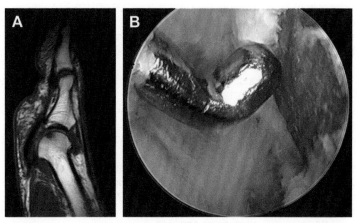

Fig. 5. (*A*) T1 sagittal MRI image demonstrating osteochondritis dessicans in the metatarsal head. (*B*) Arthroscopic image demonstrating the same osteochondritis dessicans intraoperatively.

SUMMARY

The anatomy of the first MTP joint plays a significant role in the development of hallux rigidus. Although no clear cause is identified for all cases some conclusions can be drawn from the literature regarding clinical, historical, and radiographic associations.

- Radiographic findings associated with hallux rigidus include
  - Metatarsal head OCD
  - Flattened or chevron-shaped metatarsal head
  - Elevated hallux interphalangeus angle
- Historical factors are clearly associated with hallux rigidus and should be considered when counseling patients
  - A positive family history is likely to predispose to bilateral disease
  - A positive history of trauma is likely to lead to unilateral disease
- Many clinical and radiographic findings historically suggested as etiology have been disproven in recent literature, including MPE, metatarsal length, pes planus, tight heel cords, and first ray hypermobility
- Associated anatomic findings (ie, hallux valgus, hallux valgus interphalangeus, OCD), regardless of their role in etiology, should be identified during the diagnostic evaluation of hallux rigidus; when appropriate, these findings can be addressed at the time of surgical intervention

SUPPLEMENTARY DATA

Supplementary data related to this article can be found online at http://dx.doi.org/10.1016/j.fcl.2015.04.001.

REFERENCES

1. Shurnas P, Coughlin M. Arthritic conditions of the foot, in surgery of the foot and ankle. Philadelphia: Elsevier; 2007. p. 867–909.
2. Coughlin MJ, Shurnas PS. Hallux rigidus. Grading and long-term results of operative treatment. J Bone Joint Surg Am 2003;85-A(11):2072–88.
3. Horton GA, Park YW, Myerson MS. Role of metatarsus primus elevatus in the pathogenesis of hallux rigidus. Foot Ankle Int 1999;20(12):777–80.
4. Mann RA, Coughlin MJ, Duvries HL. Hallux rigidus: a review of the literature and a method of treatment. Clin Orthopaedics Relat Res 1979;142:57–63.
5. McMaster M. The pathogenesis of hallux rigidus. J Bone Joint Surg Br 1978; 60(1):82–7.
6. Shurnas PS. Hallux rigidus: etiology, biomechanics, and nonoperative treatment. Foot Ankle Clin 2009;14(1):1–8.
7. Yee G, Lau J. Current concepts review: hallux rigidus. Foot Ankle Int 2008;29(6): 637–46.
8. Davies-Colley M. Contraction of the metatarsophalangeal joint of the great toe. BMJ 1887;1:728.
9. Cotterill J. Stiffness of the great toe in adolescents. BMJ 1888;1:1158.
10. Coughlin MJ, Shurnas PS. Hallux rigidus: demographics, etiology, and radiographic assessment. Foot Ankle Int 2003;24(10):731–43.
11. Schweitzer M, Maheshwari S, Shabshin N. Hallux valgus and hallux rigidus: MRI findings. Clin Imaging 1999;23(6):397–402.
12. Sarrafian SK. Anatomy of the foot and ankle. 2nd edition. , Philadelphia: J.B. Lippincott Company; 1993.

13. Lucas DE, Philbin T, Hatic S 2nd. The plantar plate of the first metatarsophalangeal joint: an anatomical study. Foot Ankle Spec 2014;7(2):108–12.
14. Shereff MJ, Bejjani FJ, Kummer FJ. Kinematics of the first metatarsophalangeal joint. J Bone Joint Surg Am 1986;68-A(3):392–8.
15. Drago JJ, Oloff L, Jacobs AM. A comprehensive review of hallux limitus. J Foot Surg 1984;23(3):213–20.
16. Goodfellow J. Aetiology of hallux rigidus. Proc R Soc Med 1966;59:821–4.
17. Bonney G, Macnab I. Hallux valgus and hallus rigidus. J Bone Joint Surg Br 1952; 34(3):366–85.
18. Jack E. The aetiology of hallux rigidus. Br J Surg 1940;27:492–7.
19. Klaue K, Hansen ST, Masquelet AC. Clinical, quantitative assessment of first tarsometatarsal mobility in the sagittal plane and its relation to hallux valgus deformity. Foot Ankle Int 1994;15(1):9–13.
20. Coughlin MJ, Shurnas PJ. Soft-tissue arthroplasty for hallux rigidus. Foot Ankle Int 2003;24(661):661–72.
21. Lambrinudi C. Metatarsus primus elevatus. Proc R Soc Med 1938;31(1273):51.
22. Kessel L, Bonney G. Hallux rigidus in the adolescent. J Bone Joint Surg Br 1958; 40(4):668–73.
23. Meyer JO, Nishon LR, Weiss L, et al. Metatarsus primus elevatus and the etiology of hallux rigidus. J Foot Surg 1987;26(3):237–41.
24. Hunt K, Anderson R. Biplanar proximal phalanx closing wedge osteotomy for hallux rigidus. Foot Ankle Int 2012;33(12):1043–50.
25. Bingold A, Collins D. Hallux rigidus. J Bone Joint Surg Br 1950;32(2):214–22.
26. Nilsonne H. Hallux rigidus and it's treatment. Acta Orthop Scand 1930;1:295–303.
27. Harris R, Beath T. Hypermobile flat-foot with short tendo achillis. J Bone Joint Surg Am 1948;30(1):116–50.
28. DiGiovanni C, Kuo R, Tejwani N, et al. Isolated gastrocnemius tightness. J Bone Joint Surg Am 2002;84(6):962–70.
29. Stein G, Pawel A, Koebke J, et al. Morphology of the first metatarsal head and hallux rigidus: a cadaveric study. Surg Radiol Anat 2012;34(7):589–92.

Clinical Presentation and Management of Hallux Rigidus

Kamran S. Hamid, MD, MPH[a], Selene G. Parekh, MD, MBA[b],*

KEYWORDS

- Hallux rigidus • Arthritis • Degenerative joint disease • Metatarsophalangeal joint

KEY POINTS

- Initial management of hallux rigidus should focus on reduction in pain-inducing dorsiflexion of the first metatarsophalangeal joint through altered shoewear and activity modification.
- Surgical candidacy for hallux rigidus is based on age, activity level, clinical examination, and radiographic grading of first metatarsophalangeal degenerative joint disease.
- Dorsal cheilectomy is the commonest procedure for most low- to midgrade hallux rigidus disease, and has been found to have good clinical results.
- For patients with more severe hallux rigidus, arthrodesis or arthroplasty procedures may prove beneficial depending on functional demands.

INTRODUCTION

Hallux rigidus, Latin for "stiff toe," is an osteoarthritic condition of the first metatarsophalangeal joint characterized by pain, functional limitation, and radiographic degenerative joint disease. It is the most common form of arthritis in the foot, and its incidence is increasing with an aging population.[1,2] The underlying pathology resulting in hallux rigidus has not been elucidated in the literature because of limited ability to determine temporality and causation, but correlations with various parameters have been determined: flat first metatarsophalangeal joint, hallux valgus interphalangeus, metatarsus adductus, bilaterality in individuals with a family history of hallux rigidus, history of traumatic insult to the joint, and female gender.[3,4] Historical data demonstrate wide variations in prevalence, with some evidence pointing to 10% radiographic

The authors have nothing to disclose.
[a] Department of Orthopaedic Surgery, Wake Forest School of Medicine, Winston-Salem, NC 27157, USA; [b] Department of Orthopaedic Surgery, North Carolina Orthopaedic Clinic, Duke University School of Medicine, 3609 Southwest Durham Drive, Durham, NC 27707, USA
* Corresponding author.
E-mail address: selene.parekh@gmail.com

Foot Ankle Clin N Am 20 (2015) 391–399
http://dx.doi.org/10.1016/j.fcl.2015.04.002
1083-7515/15/$ – see front matter © 2015 Elsevier Inc. All rights reserved.

foot.theclinics.com

findings of hallux rigidus in the 20- to 34 year-old age range,[5] whereas others find only 2.5% prevalence in adults older than 50 years.[6]

CLINICAL PRESENTATION

The patient with symptomatic hallux rigidus presents with a reliable constellation of signs and symptoms consistent with degeneration of the first metatarsophalangeal joint, presumably from intrinsic and/or acquired dysfunctional joint mechanics. Symptoms include decreased range of motion (ROM) and pain with extremes of motion, often pronounced during the lift-off phase of gait, and even neuritic pain with impingement of the medial branch of the superficial peroneal nerve from the dorsal osteophytes. As the first metatarsophalangeal joint progressively deteriorates to a more advanced stage of the disease, the patient is afflicted with the hallmark symptom of midrange arthralgia in addition to pain present at full dorsiflexion and plantarflexion. If not treated, the natural course of the disease results in the hallux becoming severely painful with minimal residual functional movement.[1,3,4,7]

On physical examination in the clinician's office, the patient may be noted to have a dorsally located prominence above the first metatarsophalangeal joint correlating with dorsal metatarsal head bone spur and associated inflammation (**Fig. 1**). Further examination often demonstrates swelling, tenderness to palpation, and repeatable ROM findings that parallel the pain patterns described by the patient.[1,2,8–11] In the early stages of disease, there can be pain with extremes of sagittal plane motion but minimal pain in midrange motion. Plantarflexion pain can occur from stretching of the capsule over the dorsal osteophytes and dorsiflexion pain from impingement. Minimal pain with midrange motion is referred to as a negative "grind" test, as there is likely chondral preservation in the central/plantar articular surfaces.

IMAGING

Weight-bearing anteroposterior and lateral radiographs are considered the standard for radiographic evaluation of hallux rigidus (**Fig. 2**). Sesamoid views may be helpful for grade 0 to 1 disease, but progressive stages are often too limited in dorsiflexion to permit this view. The utility of computed tomography (CT) or MRI has classically been limited only to cases with suspected osteochondral cysts or osteochondral lesions in the face of normal plain film radiography findings.[2,4,8] However, CT is increasingly being used as an adjunct to better characterize the amount of hallux

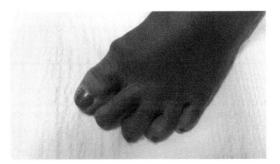

Fig. 1. Dorsally located prominence at first metatarsophalangeal joint visible on physical examination in hallux rigidus.

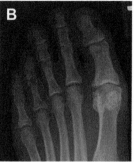
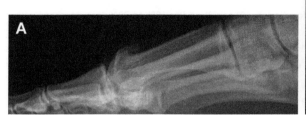

Fig. 2. (*A*) Standard weight-bearing lateral radiograph showing first metatarsophalangeal dorsal osteophytes. (*B*) Anteroposterior radiograph with evidence of joint-space narrowing.

and sesamoid osteoarthritis. This approach can drive surgical decision making from joint-sparing techniques toward fusion in severe disease.

Lateral radiographs are best suited to identify first metatarsal head dorsal osteophytosis and to track the progression of joint-space narrowing from dorsal to plantar. Anteroposterior views are considered the benchmark for assessing the joint space and evaluating the convexity of the metatarsal head. Dorsal osteophytes may obscure the view of the joint space on anteroposterior films, leading to an overestimation of osteoarthritic disease or paradoxical distraction of the joint, resulting in a false estimate of residual cartilage.[8,10] The authors consider that the interaction of sesamoid arthritis with hallux rigidus is unclear and as yet has not been sufficiently evaluated.

CLASSIFICATION

There are multitudes of classification schema that have previously been used for evaluation of hallux rigidus, including the Hattrup and Johnson, Regnauld, and Roukis classification systems.[8,12–14] During the past decade, the Coughlin and Shurnas classification of hallux rigidus has gained popularity owing to its incorporation of clinical findings (with specific parameters for passive dorsiflexion) in conjunction with established radiographic criteria. The evidence-based nature of this system aids in treatment decision making, which adds to its appeal among foot and ankle practitioners (**Box 1**).[15]

TREATMENT
Nonsurgical Management

Conservative management may provide adequate relief in appropriately selected patients, such as those with milder forms of the disease, individuals with low functional demands, and patients who are poor surgical candidates. First-line, nonoperative treatment generally consists of oral or topical nonsteroidal anti-inflammatory medications, intra-articular injection of corticosteroids or sodium hyaluronate, rigid supportive orthotics or shoewear, and lifestyle modifications. Steroid injections and nonsteroidal sodium hyaluronate injections have both demonstrated short-term benefits, although their long-term efficacy has not been validated.[16] Rigid supportive orthotics, such as a Morton Extension Footplate, extend past the first metatarsophalangeal joint, thus providing a stiff construct that allows minimal dorsiflexion at the articular surface (**Fig. 3**). Additional shoewear modifications include increasing the height and/or width of the toe box to diminish shoe rubbing against painful

---

Box 1
Clinical and radiographic classification of hallux rigidus

Grade 0

- Range of motion (ROM): dorsiflexion 40° to 60° and/or 10% to 20% loss compared with normal side
- Radiograph: normal or minimal findings
- Clinical: no subjective pain, only stiffness, loss of passive motion on examination

Grade 1

- ROM: dorsiflexion 30° to 40° and/or 20% to 50% loss compared with normal side
- Radiograph: dorsal spur is main finding; minimal joint narrowing, minimal periarticular sclerosis, minimal flattening of metatarsal head
- Clinical: mild or occasional subjective pain and stiffness, pain at extremes of dorsiflexion, and/or plantarflexion on examination

Grade 2

- ROM: dorsiflexion 10° to 30° and/or 50% to 75% loss compared with normal side
- Radiograph: dorsal, lateral, and possibly medial osteophytes give flattened appearance to metatarsal head; no more than one-fourth of dorsal joint space involvement on lateral radiograph; mild to moderate joint narrowing and sclerosis; sesamoids not usually involved but may be irregular in appearance
- Clinical: moderate to severe subjective pain and stiffness that may be constant, pain just before maximal dorsiflexion and/or plantarflexion on examination

Grade 3

- ROM: dorsiflexion of 10° or less and/or 75% to 100% loss compared with normal side, and notable loss of plantarflexion (often 10% loss).
- Radiograph: as in grade 2 but with substantial narrowing, possibly periarticular cystic changes, more than one-fourth dorsal joint may be involved on lateral radiograph, sesamoids (enlarged and/or cystic and/or irregular)
- Clinical: nearly constant subjective pain and substantial stiffness, pain throughout ROM on examination (but not at midrange)

Grade 4

- Same criteria and findings as grade 3, but definite pain at mid-ROM on examination is elicited

Data from Coughlin MJ, Shurnas PS. Hallux rigidus: grading and long-term results of operative treatment. J Bone Joint Surg Am 2003;85-A:2072–88.

---

osteophytes. Although reducing sporting or exercise activities in conjunction with altered footwear has the potential to provide substantial pain relief, these alterations may be undesirable to many active patients.[1–3,8,10,16,17]

Surgical Management

Patients on the more severe end of the disease spectrum and those refractory to conservative management may benefit from operative intervention. Surgical options can be divided into 2 distinct categories: joint-preserving and joint-altering procedures. Despite a large volume of investigative work in this arena, there remains a dearth of prospective level 1 evidence confirming the superiority of one technique over another.

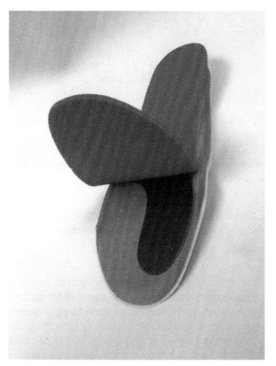

Fig. 3. Morton's extension rigid orthotic used to limit first metatarsophalangeal motion and subsequently reduce pain.

In addition, the heterogeneity of outcome measures used in the literature, small sample sizes, questions of intraobserver reliability and precision, and debatable external validity of single-surgeon studies makes this area of research less amenable to rigorous meta-analyses. For this reason, the authors describe here the basic surgical options but without presenting an exhaustive literature review beyond the scope of this article.

Joint-preserving procedures
The commonest operative technique for milder forms of hallux rigidus is the dorsal cheilectomy, a procedure that involves excision of dorsal osteophytes and partial ostectomy of the dorsal metatarsal head.[18] It is estimated that up to 30% of the dorsal metatarsal head may be excised to prevent painful impingement without leading to first metatarsophalangeal joint subluxation (**Fig. 4**).[11] By definition, dorsal cheilectomy destroys a portion of the articular surface, but because a functional majority of the surface remains unaltered, the opinion of most investigators is that it should be classified as joint preserving. The dorsal cheilectomy is often performed in tandem with procedures mitigating the effects of the proximal phalanx on dorsal impingement. Often this may entail simply excising the dorsal lip of the proximal phalanx at the first metatarsophalangeal joint, although some surgeons advocate a formal dorsal closing wedge osteotomy of the proximal phalanx (Moberg procedure) to improve baseline extension and negate the need for painful dorsiflexion. In addition, there are several metatarsal osteotomies that result in length alteration, translation, and rotational realignment of the metatarsal head, such as the Watermann, Youngswick, Reverdin Green,

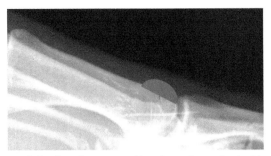

Fig. 4. Thirty percent of the dorsal metatarsal head may be excised without leading to first metatarsophalangeal joint subluxation.

Watermann Green, distal oblique sliding osteotomy, Sagittal Z osteotomy, biplanar proximal closing wedge osteotomy, and Drago procedures.[8–10,15,19,20]

Joint-altering procedures

Joint-altering procedures are ones whereby the native articulation of the first metatarsophalangeal joint is no longer maintained; they are used for patients with severe disease or those who have failed joint-preserving procedures. Arthrodesis is considered the standard of care for pain reduction in this demographic (**Fig. 5**). Surface preparation in arthrodesis involves denuding of cartilage with flat or conical molding of the metatarsal head, and creation of a complementary denuded proximal phalangeal surface. Compression and internal fixation can be achieved through multiple means including screws, staples, wires, or plates. Recommended positioning of the hallux in relation to the floor is 10° to 15° of dorsiflexion and 10° to 15° of valgus.[9,21] An excessively medialized great toe can result in friction with shoewear.[8]

Although arthrodesis is appealing because of the significant pain relief it provides, it comes with the cost of limited joint motion resulting in decreased functional capacity. Arthroplasty is a motion-preserving option with numerous choices, ranging from total metatarsophalangeal joint arthroplasty[22–28] to hemiarthroplasty[29–36] to interpositional arthroplasty,[37–39] all described with varying degrees of success. Simple resection of

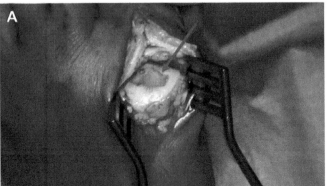
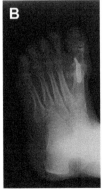

Fig. 5. (A) Intraoperative view of degenerative changes in first metatarsal head including osteophytes and articular erosion (*arrow*). (B) Anteroposterior radiograph demonstrating postoperative appearance after arthrodesis of the first metatarsophalangeal joint.

the first metatarsophalangeal articular surfaces (Keller resection arthroplasty) without replacement of the joint space with nontissue implants has also demonstrated a modicum of success in the literature.[38,40–42] As prospective studies approach the intermediate and long-term follow-up marks, the most suitable arthroplasty techniques and implants will likely become better determined.

SUMMARY

Degenerative joint disease of the first metatarsophalangeal joint is termed hallux rigidus. Hallux rigidus is the most commonly occurring arthritic condition of the foot and is marked by pain, limited motion in the sagittal plane of the first metatarsophalangeal joint, and varying degrees of functional impairment. In conjunction with clinical findings, radiographic grading helps guide therapeutic choices. The most popularly used modern grading classification is that described by Coughlin and Shurnas.[15] Nonsurgical management with anti-inflammatory medications, corticosteroid injections, or shoewear and activity modifications can be successful in appropriately selected patients. Patients with more severe disease or those refractory to conservative management may benefit from surgical intervention. Operative options range from joint-preserving procedures such as cheilectomy with or without associated osteotomies to joint-altering procedures such as arthroplasty or arthrodesis. There remains a great deal of debate in the literature regarding the efficacy of each surgical treatment option. Further well-designed clinical studies using consistent outcome measures and examining the utility of these surgical techniques, with adjustment for patient and disease severity factors, are warranted to provide valid comparisons.

REFERENCES

1. Dellenbaugh SG, Bustillo J. Arthritides of the foot. Med Clin North Am 2014;98: 253–65.
2. Iagnocco A, Rizzo C, Gattamelata A, et al. Osteoarthritis of the foot: a review of the current state of knowledge. Med Ultrason 2013;15:35–40.
3. Shurnas PS. Hallux rigidus: etiology, biomechanics, and nonoperative treatment. Foot Ankle Clin 2009;14:1–8.
4. Coughlin MJ, Shurnas PS. Hallux rigidus: demographics, etiology, and radiographic assessment. Foot Ankle Int 2003;24:731–43.
5. van Saase JL, van Romunde LK, Cats A, et al. Epidemiology of osteoarthritis: Zoetermeer survey. Comparison of radiological osteoarthritis in a Dutch population with that in 10 other populations. Ann Rheum Dis 1989;48:271–80.
6. Gould N, Schneider W, Ashikaga T. Epidemiological survey of foot problems in the continental United States: 1978–1979. Foot Ankle 1980;1:8–10.
7. Van Beek C, Greisberg J. Mobility of the first ray: review article. Foot Ankle Int 2011;32:917–22.
8. Deland JT, Williams BR. Surgical management of hallux rigidus. J Am Acad Orthop Surg 2012;20:347–58.
9. McNeil DS, Baumhauer JF, Glazebrook MA. Evidence-based analysis of the efficacy for operative treatment of hallux rigidus. Foot Ankle Int 2013;34:15–32.
10. Polzer H, Polzer S, Brumann M, et al. Hallux rigidus: joint preserving alternatives to arthrodesis - a review of the literature. World J Orthop 2014;5:6–13.
11. Seibert NR, Kadakia AR. Surgical management of hallux rigidus: cheilectomy and osteotomy (phalanx and metatarsal). Foot Ankle Clin 2009;14:9–22.
12. Hattrup SJ, Johnson KA. Subjective results of hallux rigidus following treatment with cheilectomy. Clin Orthop Relat Res 1988;(226):182–91.

13. Roukis TS, Jacobs PM, Dawson DM, et al. A prospective comparison of clinical, radiographic, and intraoperative features of hallux rigidus: short-term follow-up and analysis. J Foot Ankle Surg 2002;41:158–65.

14. Roukis TS, Jacobs PM, Dawson DM, et al. A prospective comparison of clinical, radiographic, and intraoperative features of hallux rigidus. J Foot Ankle Surg 2002;41:76–95.

15. Coughlin MJ, Shurnas PS. Hallux rigidus. Grading and long-term results of operative treatment. J Bone Joint Surg Am 2003;85-A:2072–88.

16. Pons M, Alvarez F, Solana J, et al. Sodium hyaluronate in the treatment of hallux rigidus. A single-blind, randomized study. Foot Ankle Int 2007;28:38–42.

17. Aggarwal A, Kumar S, Kumar R. Therapeutic management of the hallux rigidus. Rehabil Res Pract 2012;2012:479046.

18. Mann RA, Coughlin MJ, DuVries HL. Hallux rigidus: a review of the literature and a method of treatment. Clin Orthop Relat Res 1979;(142):57–63.

19. Bussewitz BW, Dyment MM, Hyer CF. Intermediate-term results following first metatarsal cheilectomy. Foot Ankle Spec 2013;6:191–5.

20. Hunt KJ, Anderson RB. Biplanar proximal phalanx closing wedge osteotomy for hallux rigidus. Foot Ankle Int 2012;33:1043–50.

21. Kelikian AS. Technical considerations in hallux metatarsal-phalangeal arthrodesis. Foot Ankle Clin 2005;10:167–90.

22. Becerro de Bengoa Vallejo R, Losa Iglesias ME, Jules KT. Tendon insertion at the base of the proximal phalanx of the hallux: surgical implications. J Foot Ankle Surg 2012;51:729–33.

23. Chee YH, Clement N, Ahmed I, et al. Functional outcomes following ceramic total joint replacement for hallux rigidus. Foot Ankle Surg 2011;17:8–12.

24. Dawson-Bowling S, Adimonye A, Cohen A, et al. MOJE ceramic metatarsophalangeal arthroplasty: disappointing clinical results at two to eight years. Foot Ankle Int 2012;33:560–4.

25. Duncan NS, Farrar NG, Rajan RA. Early results of first metatarsophalangeal joint replacement using the toefit-plus prosthesis. J Foot Ankle Surg 2014;53:265–8.

26. Erkocak OF, Senaran H, Altan E, et al. Short-term functional outcomes of first metatarsophalangeal total joint replacement for hallux rigidus. Foot Ankle Int 2013;34:1569–79.

27. Kim PJ, Hatch D, Didomenico LA, et al. A multicenter retrospective review of outcomes for arthrodesis, hemi-metallic joint implant, and resectional arthroplasty in the surgical treatment of end-stage hallux rigidus. J Foot Ankle Surg 2012;51:50–6.

28. Lawrence BR, Thuen E. A retrospective review of the primus first MTP joint double-stemmed silicone implant. Foot Ankle Spec 2013;6:94–100.

29. Erdil M, Bilsel K, Imren Y, et al. Metatarsal head resurfacing hemiarthroplasty in the treatment of advanced stage hallux rigidus: outcomes in the short-term. Acta Orthop Traumatol Turc 2012;46:281–5.

30. Erdil M, Elmadag NM, Polat G, et al. Comparison of arthrodesis, resurfacing hemiarthroplasty, and total joint replacement in the treatment of advanced hallux rigidus. J Foot Ankle Surg 2013;52:588–93.

31. Giza E, Sullivan M, Ocel D, et al. First metatarsophalangeal hemiarthroplasty for hallux rigidus. Int Orthop 2010;34:1193–8.

32. Konkel KF, Menger AG. Mid-term results of titanium hemi-great toe implants. Foot Ankle Int 2006;27:922–9.

33. Ronconi P, Martinelli N, Cancilleri F, et al. Hemiarthroplasty and distal oblique first metatarsal osteotomy for hallux rigidus. Foot Ankle Int 2011;32:148–52.

34. Shankar NS. Silastic single-stem implants in the treatment of hallux rigidus. Foot Ankle Int 1995;16:487–91.
35. Sorbie C, Saunders GA. Hemiarthroplasty in the treatment of hallux rigidus. Foot Ankle Int 2008;29:273–81.
36. Taranow WS, Moutsatson MJ, Cooper JM. Contemporary approaches to stage II and III hallux rigidus: the role of metallic hemiarthroplasty of the proximal phalanx. Foot Ankle Clin 2005;10:713–28, ix–x.
37. Lau JT, Daniels TR. Outcomes following cheilectomy and interpositional arthroplasty in hallux rigidus. Foot Ankle Int 2001;22:462–70.
38. Schenk S, Meizer R, Kramer R, et al. Resection arthroplasty with and without capsular interposition for treatment of severe hallux rigidus. Int Orthop 2009;33:145–50.
39. Hyer CF, Granata JD, Berlet GC, et al. Interpositional arthroplasty of the first metatarsophalangeal joint using a regenerative tissue matrix for the treatment of advanced hallux rigidus: 5-year case series follow-up. Foot Ankle Spec 2012;5:249–52.
40. Mroczek KJ, Miller SD. The modified oblique Keller procedure: a technique for dorsal approach interposition arthroplasty sparing the flexor tendons. Foot Ankle Int 2003;24:521–2.
41. Schneider W, Kadnar G, Kranzl A, et al. Long-term results following Keller resection arthroplasty for hallux rigidus. Foot Ankle Int 2011;32:933–9.
42. Brage ME, Ball ST. Surgical options for salvage of end-stage hallux rigidus. Foot Ankle Clin 2002;7:49–73.

Hallux Rigidus

Nonoperative Treatment and Orthotics

Remesh Kunnasegaran, MBChB (Glasgow), MRCS (Glasgow),
Gowreeson Thevendran, MBChB (Bristol), MFSEM (UK), FRCS Ed (Tr & Orth)*

KEYWORDS

• Hallux rigidus • Osteoarthritis • Nonoperative • Orthotics

KEY POINTS

- There is a reasonable body of evidence to substantiate the role of nonoperative management for hallux rigidus.
- At present, there is conflicting evidence for the role of manipulation and injection therapy.
- There is weak evidence to support the role of orthotics and supportive shoes for the treatment of hallux rigidus and this treatment modality may be best suited for lower grades of hallux rigidus and selected groups of patients.
- The application of newer experimental modalities, such as extracorporeal shockwave therapy, iontophoresis, and ultrasonography therapy, although increasing in popularity, has yet to be shown to be an evidence-based practice for the treatment of hallux rigidus.

INTRODUCTION

Hallux rigidus refers to degenerative arthritis of the first metatarsophalangeal joint (MTPJ). The condition was first reported by Davies-Colley[1] in 1887 who described a plantar-flexed position of the proximal phalanx in relation to the metatarsal head and coined the term hallux flexus. Cotterill[2] later described the term hallux rigidus to characterize the painful limitation of motion of the first MTPJ. Both hallux limitus and hallux rigidus are clinical and diagnostic terms that represent progressive phases in a spectrum of the same disorder with no distinct markers between the phases. DuVries[3] and Moberg[4] noted that after hallux valgus, hallux rigidus is the most common disorder affecting the first MTPJ.

Since the first publications relating to its management in the late 1880s, a wide array of options for the treatment of hallux rigidus has been discussed. Although the current

Disclosure: The authors have nothing to disclose.
Department of Orthopaedics, Tan Tock Seng Hospital, 11 Jalan Tan Tock Seng, Singapore 308433, Singapore
* Corresponding author.
E-mail address: gowreeson_thevendran@ttsh.com.sg

Foot Ankle Clin N Am 20 (2015) 401–412
http://dx.doi.org/10.1016/j.fcl.2015.04.003
1083-7515/15/$ – see front matter © 2015 Elsevier Inc. All rights reserved.

literature favors surgical intervention, considerable controversy still surrounds these procedures with regard to their indications and results. This conundrum is partly influenced by the variability in the natural history of the evolution of hallux rigidus because in some cases the condition assumes a fairly indolent course with little progression in symptoms. The ever-increasing choice of treatment options coupled with the uncertainty in outcomes renders clinical decision making challenging. This article briefly discusses the proposed cause of hallux rigidus, clinical presentation and grading, and the role of nonoperative treatment options.

CAUSE

The prevalence of hallux rigidus, as described in the available literature, has been noted to favor the female gender, with bilateral disease being more common then unilateral.[5-7] Coughlin and Shurnas[5] reviewed 110 patients, 87 of whom (79%) had bilateral disease clinically and radiographically at the final follow-up, compared with 22 of 110 patients (19%) seen at the initial examination. Of the 110 patients in their study, 74 had a positive family history and 70 of these patients had bilateral disease.[5]

The cause of hallux rigidus is not well understood, with numerous hypotheses on contributory factors postulated but with no proven association. Proposed factors include second ray metatarsal length exceeding that of the first ray, first ray hypermobility, Achilles tendon contracture, planovalgus or cavus foot posture, poor footwear, hallux valgus, functional hallux limitus, occupation, mismatch between the metatarsal head and the hemispherical articular surface of the proximal phalanx, metatarsus adductus, hallux valgus interphalangeus, and metatarsus primus elevatus.[6-10] A finite-element analysis study of the MTPJ in hallux rigidus by Flavin and colleagues[11] suggested a correlation between the increase in the tension of the plantar fascia and hallux rigidus stemming from an increase in the stress on the articular cartilage of the MTPJ. In contrast, Coughlin and Shurnas[5] found that there is no association between hallux rigidus and trauma, shoe wear, Achilles tendon tightness, or metatarsus primus elevatus. However, they did suggest a link between metatarsal head articular shape (ie, flat, chevron), metatarsal adductus, and hallux valgus interphalangeus and hallux rigidus.[5,12]

Despite the multitude of factors, the most common cause reported in the literature is trauma, either via a single isolated injury resulting in a fracture and eventually unilateral hallux rigidus[5] or chronic repetitive microtrauma.[13] A hyperextension injury to the plantar plate and sesamoid complex (so-called turf toe)[14,15] and a hyperplantar flexion injury (sand toe)[16] may create compression or shear forces that then lead to chondral or osteochondral injury, capsular damage, synovitis, and adhesions, and thus have been linked to the development of hallux rigidus.

Metatarsus primus elevatus has also been implicated as a potential causative factor in the pathogenesis of hallux rigidus. First reported by Lambrinudi[17] in 1938 who defined it as an abnormal elevation of the first ray, and subsequently called it metatarsus primus elevatus. Iatrogenic causes such as first metatarsal osteotomy or a fracture malunion may predispose to a fixed deformity. In contrast, a flexible deformity may be caused by posterior tibial tendon dysfunction, weakness of the peroneal muscles, spastic conditions, and paralysis. Several investigators have proposed correction of this anatomic abnormality as a treatment of hallux rigidus.[8] However, there are studies that describe metatarsus primus elevatus as a consequence of the arthritic progression and loss of the MTPJ range of motion.[5,12,18] Meyer and colleagues[19] found no statistically significant relationship between metatarsus primus elevatus and hallux rigidus. Myerson and colleagues[20] reviewed 264 lateral weight-bearing radiographs from 81 patients with hallux rigidus, 50 asymptomatic volunteers, and 64 patients with a diagnosis of isolated Morton neuroma. The mean elevation was 7.3 and 7.4 mm in grade I and II hallux rigidus, respectively. An average of nearly 8 mm of metatarsus primus elevatus is a normal finding. A mean elevation of 9.2 mm was noted in patients with advanced hallux rigidus. Thus, it was concluded that there was no direct or linear relationship between the elevation of the first ray and the grade of hallux rigidus. They suggested that the elevation of the first metatarsal in patients with advanced osteoarthritis of the first MTPJ is a secondary phenomenon rather than a primary causative factor.

BIOMECHANICS AND PATHOPHYSIOLOGY

The normal MTPJ has a range of motion of 110°, with a plantar flexion of 35° and dorsiflexion of 75°.[21] The consistency and three-dimensional geometry of the articular surfaces confer stability to the center of rotation of the joint, which is also stabilized by the articular capsule, the plantar fascia, the lateral ligaments, and the dynamic structures, namely the extensor hallucis longus, flexor hallucis longus, flexor hallucis brevis, hallucis abductor, and hallucis adductor.[21]

In a normal foot, the centers of rotation are constant in motion and are on the metatarsal head, but in hallux rigidus they are located outside or eccentrically to the metatarsal head.[11,21] The proximal phalanx moves gradually into a plantar position relative to the metatarsal head, resulting in progressive displacement of the center of rotation.[11] This displacement causes dorsal clamping of the joint during dorsiflexion. Cartilage lesions occur on the dorsal aspect of the first metatarsal head because of repeated compression under high stresses. This compression eventually leads to the development of dorsal osteophytes, joint degeneration, and possibly total ankylosis.

The sesamoids are also involved as a result of the retraction of the plantar structures, with a displacement of the centers of rotation and resultant articular surface compression throughout the range of motion and stiffness.[11] Sesamoid hypertrophy occurs because of an excessive continuous traction with extension in the sagittal plane.[22] Retraction of the flexor hallucis brevis can also lead to proximal displacement of the sesamoids relative to the metatarsal head.[22]

CLINICAL PRESENTATION AND GRADING

In the early stages, hallux rigidus commonly manifests as pain, particularly on the dorsal aspect; inflammation; and mild restriction in the range of motion of the first MTPJ. Flares of swelling and pain become more frequent and symptoms become more pronounced as the degeneration worsens.[23] Cartilage depletion is typically seen on the dorsal portion of the metatarsal head, with the subsequent formation of dorsal and dorsolateral osteophytes on the metatarsal head as the disease progresses.[24] These osteophytes eventually give rise to a dorsal prominence that may predispose to diffuse pain and inflammation with constant friction against the shoe. Numbness along the medial border of the hallux may result from compression of dorsomedial cutaneous nerve.[8] Activities that may aggravate the pain include those that involve increased loading on the first MTPJ, such as tiptoeing and running. Patients may also report difficulty with sustained activity while barefooted or in soft-soled shoes. Compensatory offloading of the hallux and the medial column may cause pain on the lateral aspect of the foot.[24] Patients may also complain of ipsilateral hip pain from external rotator muscle tightness secondary to lower limb external rotation.

Physical examination frequently reveals a tender, swollen MTPJ with limited range of motion. Crepitus and grinding are felt, with pain mainly elicited in dorsiflexion, plantar flexion, or both. An indication of significant cartilage loss is pain in the mid-range of motion with gentle loading. Restricted MTPJ dorsiflexion may be compensated for with interphalangeal joint hyperextension. As the MTPJ stiffens and transfer of weight to the lateral border of the foot continues, the patient's gait becomes increasingly antalgic. Transfer metatarsalgia may eventually occur and a positive Tinel sign may be elicited if there is compression of dorsomedial cutaneous nerve.[8]

RADIOLOGICAL FINDINGS AND GRADING

Standing anteroposterior, oblique, and lateral radiographs are sufficient in the evaluation of patients with hallux rigidus. Asymmetric joint space narrowing and flattened widening of the metatarsal head can be seen on the anteroposterior radiograph. Other features usually seen in the later stages of hallux rigidus include cystic changes in the metatarsal, sclerosis, formation of osteophytes at the base of the proximal phalanx, and sesamoid enlargement. The dorsal metatarsal osteophyte is often more apparent on the lateral radiograph of the foot.[8]

Several classification systems have been described for the staging of hallux rigidus clinically, radiographically, and/or intraoperatively. In 1988, hallux rigidus was classified into 3 different grades by Hattrup and Johnson.[24]

- Grade 1: mild changes with maintained joint space with minimal spurring
- Grade 2: moderate disease with joint space narrowing, bony proliferation of the metatarsal head and phalanx, and subchondral sclerosis or cyst
- Grade 3: severe hallux rigidus with severe joint space narrowing, significant bony proliferation, and loose bodies or a dorsal ossicle

A more elaborate classification system was proposed by Coughlin and Shurnas[12] in 1999, which took into consideration both clinical and radiographic parameters. It is the most comprehensive classification and is universally used (**Table 1**).

NONOPERATIVE TREATMENT OF HALLUX RIGIDUS

Most of the current literature on hallux rigidus is focused on the operative management of this condition. However, the natural history of hallux rigidus is inconsistent, with some patients reporting a more indolent course than others. In their retrospective series of patients with symptomatic hallux rigidus, Grady and colleagues[25] reviewed 772 patients who had either operative or nonoperative management. Fifty-five percent of all patients were treated successfully with conservative care alone. Of those who failed conservative treatment, 13% either refused surgery or were not surgical candidates. The investigators concluded that most patients could be treated successfully with conservative measures.

In their longitudinal questionnaire-based study of 22 consecutive patients with a minimum follow-up of 12 years, Smith and colleagues[26] evaluated the long-term outcome of patients with hallux rigidus treated nonoperatively. Only 1 patient said that his pain had worsened since his initial diagnosis, whereas 67% of patients had radiographic deterioration over time. Seventy-five percent of patients declared that they would make the same choice for nonoperative care if they had to make the same decision again. The investigators established that there was little correlation between subjective complaints and radiographic evidence of progression of hallux rigidus as manifested by loss of MTPJ space.

Various nonoperative treatment options and the current evidence for its role in the management of hallux rigidus, are discussed later.

Table 1
Coughlin and Shurnas clinical and radiographic classification of hallux rigidus

Grade	Dorsiflexion	Radiographic Findings[a]	Clinical Findings
0	40°–60° (20% loss of normal motion)	Normal	No pain. Only stiffness and loss of motion
1	30°–40° (20%–60% loss of normal motion)	Dorsal osteophyte. Minimal joint space narrowing, periarticular sclerosis and flattening of the metatarsal head	Mild or occasional pain and stiffness at the extremes of movements
2	10°–30°(50%–75% loss of normal motion)	Dorsal, lateral, and possibly medial osteophytes with flattened appearance to the metatarsal head; less than one-fourth of the dorsal joint space is involved on the lateral radiograph; mild to moderate joint space narrowing and sclerosis; sesamoids not involved	Moderate to severe pain and stiffness. Pain occurs just before maximum dorsiflexion and maximum plantar flexion
3	≤10° (75%–100% loss of normal motion). Loss of plantar flexion as well (often ≤10°)	Same as in grade 2 but with substantial narrowing, cystic changes, more than one-fourth of the dorsal joint space is involved on the lateral radiograph, sesamoids enlarged, cystic, and/or irregular	Constant pain and substantial stiffness at the extremes of range of motion but not at the midrange
4	Same as in grade 3	Same as in grade 3	Same as in grade 3 but with hindrance of passive motion

[a] Weight-bearing anteroposterior and lateral.
Adapted from Coughlin MJ, Shurnas PS. Hallux rigidus: grading and long-term results of operative treatment. J Bone Joint Surg Am 2003;85(11):2073; with permission.

Manipulation Under Anesthesia and Joint Injections

Manipulation under anesthesia (MUA) and intra-articular injection of steroids and local anesthetic have been described in the literature as a possible treatment modality. First described by Watson-Jones[27] in 1927, MUA of the first interphalangeal joint was performed with the aim of breaking down the capsular adhesions that are responsible for the flexion contracture seen in hallux rigidus. Intra-articular injection of a local anesthetic and steroids has been used as an adjunct following MUA and works by eliminating the inflammatory feedback loop.

Solan and colleagues[28] reviewed the efficacy of MUA of the first MTPJ with intra-articulation of steroids and local anesthesia in 2001. Thirty-one patients (37 MTPJs) with a diagnosis of hallux rigidus were reviewed following MUA and intra-articular injection of a mixture of 40 mg of Depo-Medrone (2 mL) made up in 3 mL of 0.5% bupivacaine. The grade of disease in each patient was determined using the Karasick and Wapner classification of radiological changes. Patients with grade 1 disease had symptomatic relief for a median period of 6 months following treatment with about one-third of patients eventually requiring surgery. In grade 2 hallux rigidus, symptomatic relief was achieved for a median period of 3 months with two-thirds of these patients ultimately requiring surgery. MUA and injection were therefore considered of limited benefit in this group of patients. Patients with grade 3 hallux rigidus had limited benefit and required surgery within 3 months of treatment. It was concluded that MUA and injection be used only in early (grades I and II) hallux rigidus.

Intra-articular injection of hyaluronan is an alternative treatment modality for patients with symptomatic hallux rigidus. Although shown to have pain-relieving properties, steroids have not been proved to slow the progression of the articular cartilage degeneration. However, hyaluronic acid has been shown to modify disease progression in various studies involving animal models, and in addition have a protective effect on articular cartilage. Studies of the knee with hyaluronic acid injections showed a reduction in the synovial inflammation, an intensification of chondrocyte density, and an improvement in the extent and degree of cartilage lesions 6 months after the injection.[29]

A randomized prospective trial by Pons and colleagues[30] in 2007 comparing intra-articular injections of steroids and hyaluronic acid in 37 patients with hallux rigidus supports the use of hyaluronic acid injections. A decrease in pain and an improvement in function in both groups of patients 3 months following the injection were shown, although pain relief was significantly better in the hyaluronic acid group. However, the study did not mention the grade or severity of the hallux rigidus in these patients and a high percentage of patients in both groups ended up requiring surgery after 1 year because of persistent pain and impaired function.[30]

Patrella and Cogliano[31] in 2003 treated 47 active golfers with hallux rigidus using intra-articular injections of hyaluronic acid. All patients had grades 1 to 3 hallux rigidus (Regnauld classification) and received weekly injections into the MTPJs for 8 weeks. The patients were evaluated at 9 weeks and 16 weeks after the first cycle of treatment, as well as at presentation for a second injection. The primary outcomes evaluated included rest pain on a visual analogue scale (VAS), MTPJ range of motion, 10-m tiptoe-walking VAS, and global patient satisfaction (GPS). There was significant improvement in rest pain, tiptoe walking pain, range of motion, and GPS for all 3 grades at 9 weeks, which was sustained at 16 weeks. Range of motion and GPS were significantly improved compared with baseline at presentation for second injection, whereas rest and tiptoe-walking VAS had returned to baseline. Adverse events were rare and included only local pain. The investigators concluded that intra-articular hyaluronic acid injections are effective and significantly improved rest and activity pain tolerance with few adverse effects.

A retrospective audit by Maher and Price[32] of 14 patients who received sodium hyaluronate injections concluded that viscosupplementation does seem to offer relief for MTPJ pain. Patients were asked to record their joint pain before and after injection using a VAS based on a 10-cm line. The average preinjection VAS score was 6.2 cm and postinjection VAS score was 2.8 cm. Duration of benefit was variable.

Munteanu and colleagues[33] concluded otherwise. In their study, 151 patients with hallux rigidus were randomized into 2 groups: with 1 group receiving hylan G-F 20 (Synvisc) and the other group receiving a placebo with normal saline. There was no statistically significant difference between the hyaluronic acid group and the placebo group with regard to pain reduction 3 months after treatment. Hyaluronic acid was therefore not recommended for the treatment of first MTPJ osteoarthritis.

Prolotherapy (short for proliferation therapy) is a term first coined by G.S. Hackett[34] in 1957 and refers to the injection of a substance that promotes growth (eg, growth factors) or substances that stimulate the production of growth factors (eg, dextrose). Animal studies have shown that prolotherapy induces collagen synthesis via the induction of an inflammatory response. Although prolotherapy use has been described in the management of hallux rigidus, the evidence for its use is weak. A retrospective observational study by Hauser and colleagues[35] in 2011 assessed 19 patients with foot and ankle pain who received 10 to 30 injections of 15% dextrose, 0.2% lidocaine, with a total of 6 to 40 mL of solution used per foot and toe, using the Hackett-Hemwall prolotherapy technique. Prolotherapy resulted in a significant decrease in pain and stiffness as well as improved quality-of-life parameters in the patients treated. However, there is currently a paucity of evidence to support the role of prolotherapy in the management of hallux rigidus and as such a treatment recommendation cannot be made.[35]

Shoe Modifications and Orthotics

Hoffmann and colleagues[36] in 1905 did a comparative study of barefooted and shoe-wearing people and noted that abnormal biomechanics of the foot may predispose to disorders of the first MTPJ and that shoes may further compound these abnormal biomechanics. Further studies have supported the idea that abnormal biomechanics of the foot may give rise to dysfunction of the MTPJ and subsequently to disorder. Shoe modifications and foot orthoses have been commonly used in treatment with the aim of modifying the biomechanics of the first MTPJs, reducing motion, limiting irritation from the dorsal osteophytes, and reducing the mechanical stresses on the joint.

An extended shank[37] is a commonly used orthosis in the management of hallux rigidus. Made of either spring steel or carbon graphite composite, these shanks are embedded between the layers of the sole, extending from the heel to the toe. Shanks can be placed in nearly any type of shoe and can be used together with a rocker sole to enhance its function. The shank also acts as a splint, preventing the shoe from bending and in the process limiting dorsiflexion of the big toe during gait and decreasing the forces acting through the midfoot and forefoot. The rocker sole is one of the most prevalent modifications, the main function of which is to rock the foot from heel strike to toe-off without requiring the shoe or foot to bend. A high toe box can also be used to prevent direct contact between the dorsal osteophyte and shoe (**Fig. 1**).[38]

The ideal foot orthosis should provide adequate shock absorption and shock attenuation, provide appropriate cushioning, redistribute weight-bearing pressures, support and splint via the total-contact concept, decrease shear, support or correct flexible deformities, limit joint motion, and accommodate fixed deformities. Foot orthoses come prefabricated or can be custom made directly from a mold of the patient's foot.

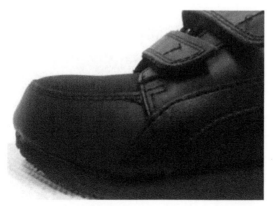

Fig. 1. Rocker bottom sole with a high toe box.

The windlass effect, as described by Hicks, involves the shortening of the plantar fascia with dorsiflexion of the hallux elevating the arch of the foot. Hicks also suggested that, if the arch of the foot were lowered, the windlass would unwind and reduce the dorsiflexion of the hallux.[39] Functional orthoses have been designed to reverse the windlass mechanism, allowing the first metatarsal to achieve sufficient plantar flexion in preparation for propulsion. Functional orthoses with a medial posting have also been fabricated with the aim of altering the degree and timing of ankle/subtalar joint complex pronation and treating first metatarsophalangeal pain. First-ray cutouts, designed to allow plantar flexion of the first ray and pronate the forefoot, and forefoot postings are other functional orthotic modifications that have been used to improve first ray function and reduce pain.[8]

In contrast, accommodative orthoses are adopted for the immobilization and for the alteration of the magnitude and temporal loading patterns of the first MTPJ. Accommodative orthoses include custom orthoses with a navicular pad and Morton extensions (**Fig. 2**).[8] Negative casts can be taken with a foam box or with plaster of Paris. A positive cast is then made from this mold to manufacture the accommodative orthoses (**Figs. 3** and **4**).

However, there are limitations in the evidence to support such treatment. Although justifiable with sound theoretic principles, the rationale for orthotic adjustment and application is currently based largely on anecdotal evidence and published case series.

Scherer and colleagues[39] studied the effect of functional foot orthoses on first metatarsophalangeal dorsiflexion and gait. Roukis[40] in 1996 established that an artificially dorsiflexed first ray in stance reduced the range of motion of the first MTPJ by 19.3%. This reduction in the dorsiflexion of the first metatarsophalangeal from dorsiflexion of the first ray has been linked to conditions such as hallux abducto valgus and hallux rigidus. Scherer and colleagues[39] proposed the use of a specific functional orthosis manufactured from a cast with the first ray plantar flexed, which raises the proximal position of the first ray and thus alters its pitch. This alteration then increased the range of dorsiflexion of the first MTPJ and simultaneously reduced the subhallux pressures. One-hundred percent of subjects showed an increase in the hallux dorsiflexion with orthoses in both stance and in gait. In stance, there was a mean increase of 8.81° or 90% in the hallux dorsiflexion.

The efficacy of modified prefabricated foot orthoses in the treatment of first metatarsophalangeal joint pain was reviewed by Welsh and colleagues.[41] Primary outcome

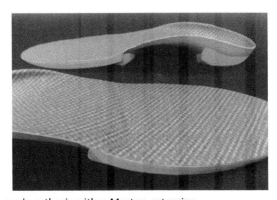

Fig. 2. A custom-made orthosis with a Morton extension.

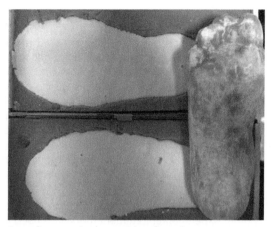

Fig. 3. The production of a negative cast with a foam box.

was pain in 32 patients with mechanical first metatarsophalangeal pain who were then provided with prefabricated foot orthoses. The investigators noted a significant decrease in first metatarsophalangeal pain between the baseline and at the 24-week end point.

In Grady and colleagues,[25] analysis of the 772 patients with symptomatic hallux limitus, 428 (55%) patients were successfully treated conservatively with 362 (84%) of these 428 patients treated with orthoses.

Physical Therapy

Physical therapy, as for most orthopedic conditions, is a major component in the treatment of hallux rigidus. Physical therapy involves joint mobilization, manipulation, improving range of motion, muscle reeducation, and strengthening of the flexor hallucis longus muscles as well as the plantar intrinsic muscles of the feet to improve the stability of the first MTPJ. Gait training, together with rest, ice, compression, and elevation, has also been advocated in the reduction of pain and inflammation.

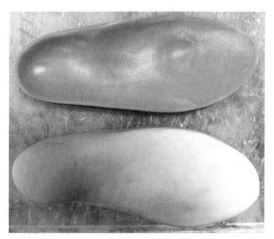

Fig. 4. Positive cast with the final product on the top.

Shamus and colleagues[42] looked at 2 conservative intervention approaches for functional hallux limitus. Twenty individuals with first MTPJ pain, stiffness, and weakness received whirlpool, ultrasonography therapy, first MTPJ mobilization, calf and hamstring stretching, marble pick-up exercises, cold packs, and electrical stimulation. The experimental group consisted of 10 of the 20 patients who further received sesamoid mobilization, flexor hallucis strengthening exercises, and gait training 3 times a week for 4 weeks. Hallux dorsiflexion, strength of the flexor hallucis longus, and subjective pain levels were assessed. After 12 therapy sessions, the experimental group achieved considerably greater MTPJ dorsiflexion and flexor hallucis longus strength and had significantly lower pain levels compared with the control group. Thus, the recommendation was for sesamoid mobilization, flexor hallucis strengthening, and gait training to be included as part of the patient' therapy regime.

Experimental Therapy

There are numerous other experimental treatment modalities used for other orthopedic conditions that have been proposed as part of the treatment armamentarium of hallux rigidus. Extracorporeal shockwave therapy has been reported as a potential treatment option and works by relieving pain by hyperstimulation analgesia and by increasing the pain threshold.[43] Animal studies have shown release of angiogenic and osteogenic growth factors in response to the shockwave therapy, resulting in tissue regeneration and repair of musculoskeletal tissue. The use of oral viscosupplementation such as glucosamine sulfate and chondroitin sulfate has also been suggested, although there is no evidence to support its specific use in the treatment of hallux rigidus.[44]

Iontophoresis, which uses electrical currents to increase absorption of topical medication within soft tissues, has been described. Ultrasonography therapy using high-frequency sound waves is also widely used in physical therapy and can be used to disintegrate scar tissue and adhesions, control the inflammatory process, and to increase soft tissue extensibility before stretching and exercises.

In summary, there is currently little evidence to support the role of these adjunct therapies in the nonoperative management of hallux rigidus.

SUMMARY

Although the literature is polarized by studies in support of operative management, there is a reasonable body of evidence to substantiate the role of nonoperative management for hallux rigidus. At present, there is conflicting evidence for the role of manipulation and injection therapy. There is weak evidence to support the role of orthotics and supportive shoes for the treatment of hallux rigidus and this treatment modality may be best suited for lower grades of hallux rigidus and selected groups of patients. There is a paucity of strong evidence to substantiate the role of physical therapy for hallux rigidus. The application of newer experimental modalities, such as extracorporeal shockwave therapy, iontophoresis, and ultrasonography therapy, although increasing in popularity, has yet to be shown to be an evidence-based practice for the treatment of hallux rigidus.

REFERENCES

1. Davies-Colley M. Contraction of the metatarsophalangeal joint of the great toe. Br Med J 1887;1:728.
2. Cotterill J. Stiffness of the great toe in adolescents. Br Med J 1888;1:1158.

3. DuVries H. Static deformities. In: DuVries H, editor. Surgery of the foot. St. Louis (MO): Mosby; 1959. p. 392–8.
4. Moberg E. A simple operation for hallux rigidus. Clin Orthop Relat Res 1979;142: 55–6.
5. Coughlin MJ, Shurnas PS. Hallux rigidus: demographics, etiology and radiographic assessment. Foot Ankle Int 2003;24:731–43.
6. Bonney G, Macnab I. Hallux valgus and hallux rigidus: a critical survey of operative results. J Bone Joint Surg Br 1952;34:366–85.
7. Drago JJ, Oloff L, Jacobs AM, et al. A comprehensive review of hallux limitus. J Foot Surg 1984;23:213–20.
8. Yee G, Lau J. Current concepts review: hallux rigidus. Foot Ankle Int 2008;29: 637–46.
9. Coughlin MJ, Mann RA, Saltzman CL. Hallux rigidus. In: Surgery of the foot and ankle. Philadelphia: Mosby-Elsevier; 2007. p. 867–921.
10. Camasta CA. Hallux limitus and hallux rigidus. Clinical examination, radiographic findings, and natural history. Clin Podiatr Med Surg 1996;13:423–48.
11. Flavin R, Halpin T, O'Sullivan R, et al. A finite-element analysis study of the metatarsophalangeal joint of the hallux rigidus. J Bone Joint Surg Br 2008;90(10):1334–40.
12. Coughlin MJ, Shurnas PS. Hallux rigidus: grading and long-term results of operative treatment. J Bone Joint Surg Am 2003;85(11):2072–88.
13. Coughlin MJ. Conditions of the forefoot. In: DeLee J, Drez D, editors. Orthopaedic sports medicine: principles and practice. Philadelphia: WB Saunders; 1994. p. P221–44.
14. Goodfellow J. Aetiology of hallux rigidus. Proc R Soc Med 1966;59:821–4.
15. McMaster MJ. The pathogenesis of hallux rigidus. J Bone Joint Surg Br 1978;60B: 82–7.
16. Frey C, Andersen GD, Feder KS, et al. Plantarflexion injury to the metatarsophalangeal joint ("sand toe"). Foot Ankle Int 1996;17:576–81.
17. Lambrinudi P. Metatarsus primus elevatus. Proc R Soc Med 1938;31:1273.
18. Coughlin MJ, Shurnas PS. Soft-tissue arthroplasty for hallux rigidus. Foot Ankle Int 2003;24:661–72.
19. Meyer JO, Nishon LR, Weiss L, et al. Metatarsus primus elevatus and the etiology of hallux rigidus. J Foot Surg 1987;26(30):237–41.
20. Horton GA, Park YW, Myerson MS. Role of metatarsus primus elevatus in the pathogenesis of hallux rigidus. Foot Ankle Int 1999;20(12):777–80.
21. Shereff MJ, Bejjani FJ, Kummer FJ. Kinematics of the first metatarsophalangeal joint. J Bone Joint Surg Am 1986;68:392–8.
22. Munuera PV, Domínguez G, Lafuente G. Length of the sesamoids and their distance from the metatarsophalangeal joint space in feet with incipient hallux limitus. J Am Podiatr Med Assoc 2008;98:123–9.
23. Shurnas PS. Hallux rigidus: etiology, biomechanics, and non-operative treatment. Foot Ankle Clin 2009;14(1):1–8.
24. Hattrup SJ, Johnson KA. Subjective results of hallux rigidus following treatment with cheilectomy. Clin Orthop Relat Res 1998;226:182–91.
25. Grady JF, Axe TM, Zager EJ, et al. A retrospective analysis of 772 patients with hallux limitus. J Am Podiatr Med Assoc 2002;92(2):102–8.
26. Smith RW, Katchis SD, Ayson LC. Outcomes in hallux rigidus patients treated nonoperatively: a long-term followup study. Foot Ankle Int 2000;21(11):906–13.
27. Watson-Jones R. Treatment of hallux rigidus [letter]. BMJ 1927;1:1165–6.
28. Solan MC, Calder JD, Bendall SP. Manipulation and injection for hallux rigidus. Is it worthwhile? J Bone Joint Surg Br 2001;83:706–8.

29. Frizziero L, Govoni E, Bacchini P. Intra-articular hyaluronic acid in the treatment of osteoarthritis of the knee: clinical and morphological study. Clin Exp Rheumatol 1998;16:441–9.

30. Pons M, Alvarez F, Solana J, et al. Sodium hyaluronate in the treatment of hallux rigidus. A single-blind randomized study. Foot Ankle Int 2005;26:1033–7.

31. Patrella RJ, Cogliano A. Intra-articular hyaluronic acid treatment for golfer's toe. Keeping older golfers on course. Phys Sportsmed 2004;32(7):41–5.

32. Maher A, Price M. An audit of the use of sodium hyaluronate 1% (Ostenil Mini [R]) therapy for the conservative treatment of hallux rigidus. Br J Podiatry 2007;10: 47–51.

33. Munteanu SE, Zammit GV, Menz HB, et al. Effectiveness of intra-articular hyaluronan (Synvisc, hylan G-F 20) for the treatment of first metatarsophalangeal joint osteoarthritis: a randomised placebo-controlled trial. Ann Rheum Dis 2011; 70(10):1838–41.

34. Hackett G. Referral pain and sciatica in diagnosis of low back disability. J Am Med Assoc 1957;163:183–5.

35. Hauser RA, Hauser MA, Cukla JK. A retrospective observational study on Hackett-Hemwall Dextrose Prolotherapy for unresolved foot and toe pain at an outpatient charity clinic in rural Illinois. J Prolotherapy 2011;3:543–51.

36. Hoffmann P. The feet of barefooted and shoe-wearing peoples. J Bone Joint Surg Am 1905;23(2):105–36.

37. Sammarco VJ, Nichols R. Orthotic management for disorders of the hallux. Foot Ankle Clin 2005;10(1):191–209.

38. Janisse DJ, Janisse E. Shoe modification and the use of orthoses in the treatment of foot and ankle pathology. J Am Acad Orthop Surg 2008;16(3):152–8.

39. Scherer PR, Sanders J, Eldredge DE, et al. Effect of functional foot orthoses on first metatarsophalangeal joint dorsiflexion in stance and gait. J Am Podiatr Med Assoc 2006;96(6):474–81.

40. Roukis TS, Scherer PR, Anderson CF. Position of the first ray and motion of the first metatarsophalangeal joint. JAPMA 1996;86:538.

41. Welsh BJ, Redmond AC, Chockalingam N, et al. A case-series study to explore the efficacy of foot orthoses in treating first metatarsophalangeal joint pain. J Foot Ankle Res 2010;3:17.

42. Shamus J, Shamus E, Gugel RN, et al. The effect of sesamoid mobilization, flexor hallucis strengthening, and gait training on reducing pain and restoring function in individuals with hallux limitus: a clinical trial. J Orthop Sports Phys Ther 2004; 34(7):368–76.

43. Ogden J, Tóth-Kischkat A, Shultheiss R. Principles of shock wave therapy. Clin Orthop 2001;387:8–17.

44. Felson DT, Lawrence RC, Hochberg MC, et al. Osteoarthritis: new insights. Part 2: treatment approaches. Ann Intern Med 2000;133:726–37.

First Metatarsophalangeal Joint Degeneration

Arthroscopic Treatment

Timo Schmid, MD[a], Alastair Younger, MD, FRCSC[b],*

KEYWORDS

- Hallux rigidus • First metatarsophalangeal degeneration • Arthroscopic debridement
- Arthroscopic fusion

KEY POINTS

- Arthroscopic treatment of hallux rigidus is appropriate after failed nonoperative treatment.
- Debridement with cheilectomy, and fusion are the main indications for arthroscopic treatment of hallux rigidus.
- If the cartilage damage is extensive and the patient has consented, then a fusion is performed at the same sitting.

INTRODUCTION

Although numerous causes have been proposed for hallux rigidus, its exact cause has yet to be elucidated. Several biomechanical and structural factors have been suggested. These factors include metatarsus primus elevatus,[1] a long[2,3] or a short[4,5] metatarsal, hypermobility of the first ray,[6,7] pronation, hallux valgus,[8,9] metatarsus adductus, and Achilles or gastrocnemius tendon tightness.[7] In addition, shoe wear and occupation might play a role in the development of hallux rigidus. However, studies have failed to prove a clear relationship between these factors and osteoarthritis of the first metatarsophalangeal (MTP) joint.[10–13]

Coughlin and Shurnas[14] identified a correlation between bilateral hallux rigidus and hallux valgus interphalangeus, MTP joint shape, female gender, and a positive family history.

The authors have no direct conflicts with the topic of this article. Dr A. Younger is a consultant for Wright Medical, Acumed, and Cartiva. Dr A. Younger receives research support from Acumed, Zimmer, Bioventus, Aminox, and Cartiva.

[a] University of British Columbia, 139 Drake Street, Vancouver, BC V6Z 2T8, Canada;
[b] Department of Orthopaedics, University of British Columbia, 560 1144 Burrard Street, Vancouver, British Columbia V6Z 2A5, Canada
* Corresponding author.
E-mail addresses: ayounger@providencehealth.bc.ca; asyounger@shaw.ca

Nilsonne[2] classified hallux rigidus into 2 distinct age groups. He considered the adolescent form a primary deformity, whereas the adult form would be a secondary deformity resulting from the development of degenerative arthritis. However, Bingold and Collins[7] proposed that the 2 entities were simply a continuum of the same degenerative process. Similarly, Coughlin and Shurnas[14] found no evidence to support a requirement for a distinction based on age.

Goodfellow[15] and McMaster[16] were the first to describe acute or chronic trauma as a cause for hallux rigidus. Goodfellow reported 3 patients with osteochondral lesions of the metatarsal articular surface. Subsequently, McMaster described 7 patients with similar findings. He also demonstrated consistent histologic changes to be a cleavage of articular cartilage with detachment from, but not involvement of, subchondral bone. Therefore, he proposed the term chondritis dissecans.[16] Both suggested that adolescent hallux rigidus is a condition secondary to osteochondritis dissecans of the first metatarsal head; this seems to particularly hold true for unilateral hallux rigidus.[14]

At the authors' institution, operative procedures after failed nonoperative treatment include debridement, cheilectomy, fusion, and resection arthroplasties in selected cases. In addition, the authors' institution is involved in a prospective randomized trial evaluating the effectiveness of a new polyvinyl alcohol implant (Cartiva) to treat contained cartilage defects of the first metatarsal head.

Of the aforementioned operations, debridement, cheilectomy, and fusion can be done arthroscopically.

FIRST METATARSOPHALANGEAL ARTHROSCOPY

The first author to describe MTP arthroscopy was Watanabe in 1972.[17] However, it was not until after various authors described the technique[18–20] in the 1990s that the procedure gained clinical importance.

Since then, treatment of various pathologic abnormalities is described in literature including removal of pigmented villonodular synovitis, degenerative disease with early osteophytosis, chondromalacia, osteochondral defects, loose bodies, arthrofibrosis, synovitis, gouty arthritis,[21] medial sesamoidectomy,[22] excision of a recurrent ganglion,[23] hallux valgus,[24,25] and EHL (extensor hallucis longus) lengthening.[26]

Concerning arthroscopic treatment of hallux rigidus, Iqbal and Chana[27] reported 15 arthroscopic dorsal cheilectomies in 1998 with rapid recovery and rehabilitation, maintained pain relief, and good metatarsophalangeal joint power and motion.

Davies and Saxby[28] published the first outcome series of arthroscopic debridement in 1999 with no or minimal pain, decreased swelling, and an increased range of movement of the affected joint after a mean follow-up of 19 months.

A second case series with 19 of 20 patients becoming pain free after debridement of various intra-articular pathologic abnormalities was reported in 2006.[21]

In 1998, van Dijk and colleagues[19] reported a prospective study enrolling 24 consecutive patients including 17 high-level athletes treated arthroscopically for different pathologic abnormalities. Pain, swelling, sports, and work involvements were recorded. There was one persistent loss of sensitivity of the hallux. Although 8 of 12 patients after removing dorsally located osteophytes and 3 of 4 patients treated for osteochondritis dissecans showed good or excellent results, results after sesamoid bone removal and treatment of hallux rigidus were less favorable.[19]

The usually stated benefits of arthroscopic procedures compared with open procedures are reduction of wound complications, faster rehabilitation, and shorter hospital stays. Arthroscopic ankle fusion was shown to be superior to open fusion regarding ankle osteoarthritis scores after 1- and 2-year follow-up.[29] To date, no studies comparing arthroscopic with open hallux rigidus operations are available. However, in the authors' experience, patients may have less swelling and faster recovery after arthroscopic first MTP fusion as compared with open fusion.

Indications

Dorsal osteophytes amenable to cheilectomy
Osteochondral defects amenable to debridement
Symptomatic advanced degeneration of the first MTP joint

Contraindications

Osteophytes blocking access (relative)
Bone loss or deformity requiring plate fixation for fusion

Preoperative Planning

1. Standing anterioposterior (AP) and lateral views: alignment, orientation of osteophytes (**Fig. 1**)
2. MRI (optional): beneficial for assessment of cartilage, joint capsule
3. Computed tomography (optional) to assess bony anatomy
4. For consent: possible change to an open procedure or a fusion should be added

SETUP AND SURGICAL TECHNIQUE

Preferably general or spinal anesthetic in combination with a thigh tourniquet is installed. Alternatively, with a popliteal nerve block, a calf tourniquet can be used. However, this might cause tightness of the flexor hallucis longus and flexor digitorum longus, impeding distraction of the MTP joint. In some cases, experienced surgeons

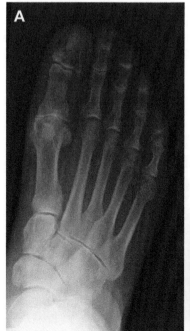
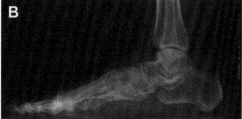

Fig. 1. AP (*A*) and lateral view (*B*) of a patient with end-stage arthritis of the first MTP joint.

can perform MTP arthroscopy under local anesthetic without using a tourniquet because Zaidi and colleagues[30] showed that ankle arthroscopy could be performed reliably without tourniquet.

The patient is placed in the supine decubitus position with a beanbag under the ipsilateral buttock to ascertain an upright position of the foot. The surgeon sits at the bottom of the bed, and the scope tower is next to the head of the bed on the opposite side of the bed to the operative limb to ensure easy visibility of the monitor during the procedure (**Fig. 2**).

Flexing and extending the joint with one hand helps to palpate the joint line with one finger of the other hand. A 6-gauge needle is placed dorsally into the joint, either medial or lateral to the extensor tendon, and the c-arm is used to confirm proper intra-articular positioning. To avoid damage to the dorsal lateral digital nerves, the portals need to be placed slightly plantar, and the incision is limited to the skin while a blunt instrument is used for deep dissection through the capsule. To prevent cartilage damage, a small cannula is inserted using a blunt probe. A 1.9-mm or 2.4-mm scope is used and preferably placed dorsomedially while placing the instruments dorsolaterally. Use of a c-arm is helpful in entering the joint on confirming the proper placement of the instruments in the joint.

If desired, a finger trap can be used to apply continuous traction. By pulling the toe with the hand and placing a blunt instrument into the joint, specific areas of the joint can be visualized in different positions of flexion and extension and the sesamoid articulation with the metatarsal head can be visualized.

Often the synovium dorsally and in the medial and lateral gutter has to be resected using the shaver to improve visualization of the joint.

In a mild hallux rigidus, a chondral defect is usually found dorsally or centrally at the basis of the phalanx or dorsally at the metatarsal head, while the subchondral bone usually remains intact. Two parallel K-wires are inserted from proximally to distally to guide the cheilectomy (**Figs. 3** and **4**). The bone resection is carried out alongside these K-wires using a lightning burr or a small osteotome (**Figs. 5** and **6**). Small residual chondral defects after cheilectomy are debrided and drilled. Remaining defects larger than 50 mm^2 and subchondral cysts are significant predictors of unsatisfactory

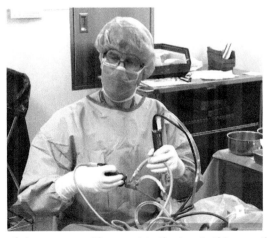

Fig. 2. Positioning of the surgeon with respect to the toe. In this case, the 2.9 arthroscope was used, but the 2.4 arthroscope may be easier to maneuver.

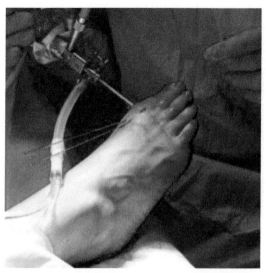

Fig. 3. Placement of the K-wires to outline the extent of the dorsal resection for a cheilectomy. The wire positions are confirmed on the c-arm. The positions of the tips of the wires are confirmed on arthroscopy to be at the edge of the cartilage rim. Two wires assist in the correct orientation of the resection. In this case, the 2.4 arthroscope is used.

clinical outcomes[31] after drilling of the metatarsal head, and a fusion might be appropriate in these cases.

Severe cases with substantial cartilage defects and sesamoid involvement are prone to failure after cheilectomy and debridement. If the patient gave consent, fusion is carried out in the same procedure. Straight and bent curettes and the shaver are used to completely remove the cartilage from the joint, and the subchondral bone is drilled using a 2.0-mm drill. After transfixation with a K-wire in appropriate position

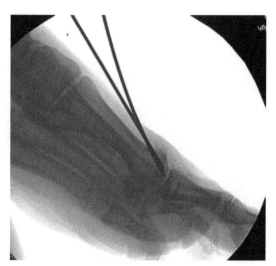

Fig. 4. Confirmation of position of the K-wires on c-arm.

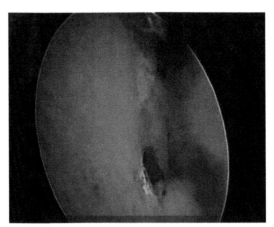

Fig. 5. The view of the tips of the K-wires from the arthroscope penetrating at the cartilage margin.

and confirming adequate bone-to-bone contact by the c-arm, 2 to 4 crossed fully threaded 3.5-mm screws are placed percutaneously to properly fix the joint.

After completion of the procedure, the tourniquet is deflated, possible bleeding is controlled, the wounds are closed with 3-0 nylon suture, and a dressing is applied.

Postoperatively, 1 to 2 weeks of non-weight-bearing suffices to allow wound healing and prevent formation of a sinus by joint fluid extravasation.

After a cheilectomy and debridement, the patient is then allowed to return to full weight-bearing in regular shoes.

After fusion, a walker boot or a shoe with a stiff sole is used to immobilize the fusion site for another 8 weeks. With this protection, weight-bearing as tolerated is allowed. Radiographs are performed at 6 and 12 weeks (**Fig. 7**), and return to sports is allowed at 4 months.

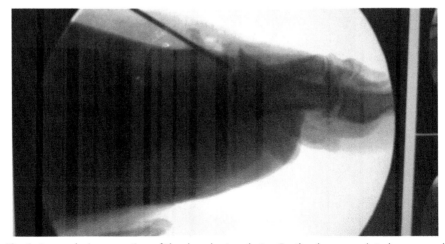

Fig. 6. Image during resection of the dorsal osteophytes. Further bone needs to be removed to complete the resection.

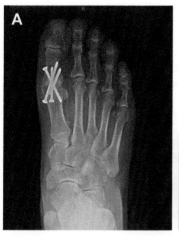
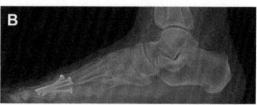

Fig. 7. Anterior posterior (*A*) and lateral views (*B*) of the case in **Fig. 1** after arthroscopic fusion and percutaneous screw placement.

SUMMARY

The arthroscopic technique allows better assessment of the cartilage surface and the ability to salvage the joint successfully. Before surgery, debridement or fusion at the time of surgery is discussed. If the joint can be salvaged, then the dorsal osteophyte excision is performed using the technique described. If the cartilage damage is extensive and the patient has consented, then a fusion is performed at the same sitting by debriding the residual cartilage and placing 3 to 4 percutaneous screws to hold the joint in a neutral position until fused.

REFERENCES

1. Lambrinudi C. Metatarsus primus elevatus. Proc R Soc Med 1938;31(11):1273.
2. Nilsonne H. Hallux rigidus and its treatment. Acta Orthop 1930;1(1–4):295–303.
3. Smith NR. Hallux valgus and rigidus treated by arthrodesis of the metatarsophalangeal joint. Br Med J 1952;2(4799):1385–7.
4. Chang TJ. Stepwise approach to hallux limitus. A surgical perspective. Clin Podiatr Med Surg 1996;13(3):449–59.
5. Kurtz DH, Harrill JC, Kaczander BI, et al. The Valenti procedure for hallux limitus: a long-term follow-up and analysis. J Foot Ankle Surg 1999;38(2):123–30.
6. Jack E. The aetiology of hallux rigidus. Br J Surg 1940;27(107):492–7.
7. Bingold AC, Collins DH. Hallux rigidus. J Bone Joint Surg Br 1950;32-B(2):214–22.
8. Lundeen RO, Rose JM. Sliding oblique osteotomy for the treatment of hallux abducto valgus associated with functional hallux limitus. J Foot Ankle Surg 2000;39(3):161–7.
9. Schweitzer ME, Maheshwari S, Shabshin N. Hallux valgus and hallux rigidus: MRI findings. Clin Imaging 1999;23(6):397–402.
10. Cracchiolo A 3rd, Weltmer JB Jr, Lian G, et al. Arthroplasty of the first metatarsophalangeal joint with a double-stem silicone implant. Results in patients who have degenerative joint disease failure of previous operations, or rheumatoid arthritis. J Bone Joint Surg Am 1992;74(4):552–63.

11. Ettl V, Radke S, Gaertner M, et al. Arthrodesis in the treatment of hallux rigidus. Int Orthop 2003;27(6):382–5.
12. O'Doherty DP, Lowrie IG, Magnussen PA, et al. The management of the painful first metatarsophalangeal joint in the older patient. Arthrodesis or Keller's arthroplasty? J Bone Joint Surg Br 1990;72(5):839–42.
13. Keogh P, Nagaria J, Stephens M. Cheilectomy for hallux rigidus. Ir J Med Sci 1992;161(12):681–3.
14. Coughlin MJ, Shurnas PS. Hallux rigidus: demographics, etiology, and radiographic assessment. Foot Ankle Int 2003;24(10):731–43.
15. Goodfellow J. Aetiology of hallux rigidus. Proc R Soc Med 1966;59(9):821–4.
16. McMaster MJ. The pathogenesis of hallux rigidus. J Bone Joint Surg Br 1978; 60(1):82–7.
17. Watanabe M. Selfoc-arthroscopy (Watanabe no 24 arthroscope) monograph. Tokyo (Japan): Teishin Hospital; 1972.
18. Ferkel RD. Arthroscopic surgery. In: Whipple TA, editor. The foot and ankle. Philadelphia: Lippincott-Raven; 1996.
19. van Dijk CN, Veenstra KM, Nuesch BC. Arthroscopic surgery of the metatarsophalangeal first joint. Arthroscopy 1998;14(8):851–5.
20. Shonka TE. Metatarsal phalangeal joint arthroscopy. J Foot Surg 1991;30(1): 26–8.
21. Debnath UK, Hemmady MV, Hariharan K. Indications for and technique of first metatarsophalangeal joint arthroscopy. Foot Ankle Int 2006;27(12):1049–54.
22. Perez Carro L, Echevarria Llata JI, Martinez Agueros JA. Arthroscopic medial bipartite sesamoidectomy of the great toe. Arthroscopy 1999;15(3):321–3.
23. Nishikawa S, Toh S. Arthroscopic treatment of a ganglion of the first metatarsophalangeal joint. Arthroscopy 2004;20(1):69–72.
24. Lui TH. First metatarsophalangeal joint arthroscopy in patients with hallux valgus. Arthroscopy 2008;24(10):1122–9.
25. Siclari A, Decantis V. Arthroscopic lateral release and percutaneous distal osteotomy for hallux valgus: a preliminary report. Foot Ankle Int 2009;30(7):675–9.
26. Lui TH. Arthroscopically assisted Z-lengthening of extensor hallucis longus tendon. Arch Orthop Trauma Surg 2007;127(9):855–7.
27. Iqbal MJ, Chana GS. Arthroscopic cheilectomy for hallux rigidus. Arthroscopy 1998;14(3):307–10.
28. Davies MS, Saxby TS. Arthroscopy of the first metatarsophalangeal joint. J Bone Joint Surg Br 1999;81(2):203–6.
29. Townshend D, Di Silvestro M, Krause F, et al. Arthroscopic versus open ankle arthrodesis: a multicenter comparative case series. J Bone Joint Surg Am 2013;95(2):98–102.
30. Zaidi R, Hasan K, Sharma A, et al. Ankle arthroscopy: a study of tourniquet versus no tourniquet. Foot Ankle Int 2014;35(5):478–82.
31. Kim YS, Park EH, Lee HJ, et al. Clinical comparison of the osteochondral autograft transfer system and subchondral drilling in osteochondral defects of the first metatarsal head. Am J Sports Med 2012;40(8):1824–33.

Open, Arthroscopic, and Percutaneous Cheilectomy for Hallux Rigidus

 CrossMark

Richard Walter, FRCS (Orth)[a], Anthony Perera, MBChB, FRCS (Orth)[b],*

KEYWORDS

- Hallux rigidus • Cheilectomy • Arthroscopic • Percutaneous • Minimally invasive

KEY POINTS

- The important factors in choosing a cheilectomy are the patient's functional expectations and the clinical examination.
- Radiographs are important for surgical planning.
- If the severity of the joint wear is unclear, then MRI can be helpful; but if this is a doubt, then arthroscopic assessment is useful.
- Thorough washout of the joint debris is key to the success of minimally invasive cheilectomy.

INTRODUCTION

Hallux rigidus is a degenerative condition of the first metatarsophalangeal (MTP) joint resulting in stiffness and pain. Typically the exostosis is found at the dorsal aspect of the distal metatarsal and proximal phalanx, resulting in painful limitation of dorsiflexion. This condition is generally primarily central on the dorsal aspect of the joint but can be more prominent medially instead, and occasionally, patients present complaining of a bunion; a historic name for this condition was dorsal bunion. In contrast to a true bunion, pain on palpation is over the dorsal joint line and especially laterally where there may be a small synovitic lesion that can be tender even in the early stages. The finding of limitation of dorsiflexion and impingement pain at the end of dorsiflexion range is classical. However, there may also be dorsal stretch pain on plantarflexion.

A wide range of management options exist, including use of rigid-soled or rocker bottom footwear, intra-articular steroid injection, cheilectomy, dorsiflexion osteotomy (of the metatarsal or proximal phalanx), interposition or implant arthroplasty, and arthrodesis. Cheilectomy is a conservative surgical option consisting of excision of

---

The authors have nothing to disclose.
[a] North Bristol NHS Trust, Bristol, BS10 5NB, UK; [b] Foot and Ankle Clinic, Spire Cardiff Hospital, Croescadarn Road, Cardiff, CF23 8XI, UK
* Corresponding author.
E-mail address: footandanklesurgery@gmail.com

the dorsal exostosis and part of the metatarsal head, with the aim of improving comfort and range of dorsiflexion. It is typically performed for patients in the earlier stages of hallux rigidus presenting with dorsal pain and dorsiflexion stiffness in the absence of through-range symptoms, rest pain, and plantar pain and with negative results on grind test.

This article describes the surgical technique and published results of isolated cheilectomy, including arthroscopic and percutaneous techniques, which have been developed with the aim of improving patient satisfaction and shortening recovery time.

Evaluation for Minimal Access Joint-Preserving Surgery

There are 3 questions to be answered:

1. Is joint-preserving surgery appropriate?
2. If so, can this be done with a minimal access approach?
3. If so, is it better done percutaneously or arthroscopically?

Radiographic scoring systems for hallux rigidus exist, and they are reasonably reproducible; however, they do not correlate well with the potential for joint-preserving surgery and are not necessarily predictive of outcome.[1] As long as there is no significant bone loss, cheilectomy can be considered even if radiographs show advanced degeneration, particularly if motion is important or if there is a short first metatarsal; however, patients should be made aware that the outcomes are reduced if the radiologic appearances are advanced. Nonetheless, some caution should be taken in selecting patients for joint-preserving surgery if there is widespread bone-on-bone degeneration. In the senior author's (Dr. Perera) experience the exception to this rule is in the case in which the primary complaint is rubbing of footwear on a large osteophyte rather than joint/impingement pain. In these cases, it is the authors' experience that patients respond well to percutaneous but not arthroscopic cheilectomy, as the arthroscopic approach requires a more significant approach in these cases.

All cheilectomy techniques regardless of the approach aim to remove only the osteophyte and the dorsal third of the metatarsal head; degeneration below this level is not removed. Although microfracture to central/inferior loss is technically possible, cartilage loss in this area has a negative effect on the outcome. One of the failings in plain-film radiographs is that they do not give a good idea of the site and size of the cartilage loss. For these reasons the fundamental decision on whether to perform joint-preserving surgery is based on clinical history and examination. It is taken that night pain and resting pain are negative prognostic factors and that fusion is a more reliable option in these situations. Plantar pain suggests inferior degeneration or metatarsosesamoid degeneration; cheilectomy does not improve this and may even make it worse. A positive result on grind test of the MTP joint or a complaint of deep pain suggests inferior spread of the degeneration, and cheilectomy is not indicated. A useful clinical test is to assess compression plantarflexion from the point of maximal dorsiflexion down to maximal plantarflexion. If this is smooth and pain-free through this arc of motion, then this cartilage is likely to be in good condition.

Findings on plain radiographs often appear worse than one would expect clinically, and this is not necessarily reason to avoid cheilectomy. In contrast, when the radiographs show little or no degeneration or dorsal osteophytosis, this is cause for caution as the degeneration is not following the typical pattern, and MRI is useful in evaluating the severity and the site of joint degeneration and may frequently reveal a central or inferior pattern of wear. This evaluation is important particularly when percutaneous cheilectomy is considered, as this is the one approach in which one does not directly visualize the joint during surgery and therefore this can be useful in decision making for the joint that on the radiograph looks either worse than expected or better than expected.

A long-standing severely stiff joint does not start moving more after cheilectomy. However, if a tip-toe lateral radiograph shows gaping on the plantar aspect compared with the plantigrade lateral view, this suggests hinging on the dorsal osteophyte with the soft-tissue potential for movement, and this may improve after cheilectomy (**Fig. 1.**)

Radiographs are, however, useful for planning the focus and extent of the excision. One can assess the size of the osteophyte and the resection required, the presence and location of loose bodies, and especially the presence of a lateral spur or a flattened metatarsal head, as these are not routinely addressed in percutaneous cheilectomy and may require accessory portals. This assessment also enables one to plan the areas that require focus during the procedure; even with arthroscopic cheilectomy it is difficult to get a global overview compared with open surgery.

OPEN CHEILECTOMY
Surgical Technique

After spinal or general anesthesia, limb exsanguination, and pneumatic thigh tourniquet inflation, a dorsomedial longitudinal incision is made, extending 3 cm distal and proximal to the first MTP joint, taking care to avoid damage to the dorsomedial cutaneous branch of the superficial peroneal nerve. The incision runs parallel and just medial to the extensor hallucis longus (EHL) tendon; in this area between the dorsal medial cutaneous nerve and the EHL tendon, there are no tendons other than the occasional accessory EHL tendon in approximately 10% of patients. Therefore, it is possible to cut directly down onto bone to minimize skin handling and trauma. For this reason, fixed retraction is to be avoided; mini Homan retractors can be used alongside the metatarsal head, retracting the deeper tissues intermittently and avoiding pulling too hard. A longitudinal dorsal capsulotomy is performed, and if there is

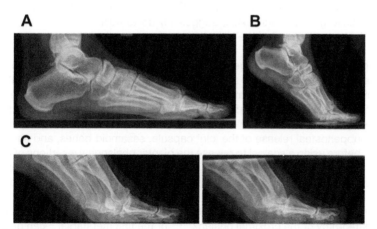

Fig. 1. (*A*) Lateral radiograph showing marked hallux rigidus; note the metatarsus elevates and blocks the free excursion of the phalanx and the plantarflexed posture of the toe. (*B*) Despite the marked degeneration, dorsiflexion is present and the dorsal impingement with plantar gapping can be seen, thus cheilectomy is likely to be successful. (*C*) A preoperative image (*i*) shows dorsal impingement and a 6-week postoperative image (*ii*) shows improved dorsal range of motion after removal of the dorsal 30% of the metatarsal head and the absence of impingement.

severe stiffness, the collateral ligaments can be released, allowing one to mobilize the sesamoid apparatus using a rounded blunt instrument. However, this increases the surgical insult and increases swelling, pain, and formation of scar tissue. As these joints are stiff, there are no concerns about the development of a deformity from this release.

Hypertrophied synovium and loose bodies are excised, and the MTP articular surface is carefully examined. If arthrosis affects greater than 50% of the joint, arthrodesis is considered. A rongeur is used to remove the osteophytes from the dorsum of the base of the first proximal phalanx. Subsequent plantarflexion exposes the metatarsal head and allows removal of the osteophytes along with the dorsal 25% of the metatarsal head, using an osteotome or small saw in a distal to proximal direction. Care is taken to not extend the resection into the diaphysis, to avoid fracture. Medial and lateral osteophytes are removed and the head rounded off, taking care not to damage the collateral ligaments. Bone wax is applied to cut bone surfaces to avoid bleeding. Dorsiflexion of 70° should be achieved intraoperatively. Manipulation of the head into forced dorsiflexion helps to mobilize and stretch the plantar tissues. It may also be necessary to remove osteophytes or even just part of the dorsal lip of the proximal phalanx to further improve the range of motion and reduce impingement.

The remaining joint surface and the metatarsal-sesamoid joints are examined for chondral erosions, which are treated with drilling with a fine Kirschner wire to promote fibrocartilage production. The joint capsule is closed deep to the EHL tendon and an absorbable subcuticular suture is used to appose the skin edges. Early full-weight-bearing mobilization is encouraged, and range of motion exercises are increased once the wound has healed at 2 weeks postoperatively.

Technical Variations

The amount of metatarsal head that should be excised is a matter of debate: some researchers recommend a conservative resection of the dorsal 15% to 20% of the articular surface, warning that exceeding this risks dorsal instability and a jerking movement during great toe dorsiflexion.[2,3] Others advocate a more generous resection to achieve greater dorsiflexion, suggesting up to 40% resection[4,5] or an even more radical resection called the Valenti procedure, a radical V-excision of the MTP joint.[6,7]

To improve the achieved range of dorsiflexion, plantar soft-tissue release can be performed. Gould[8] describes the use of a Freer elevator to clear soft-tissue adhesions on the plantar aspect of the metatarsal and to release the proximal end of the plantar plate. Thermann and Becher[2] support a more aggressive soft-tissue release, passing a McGlamry elevator proximally along the plantar aspect of the first metatarsal to achieve subperiosteal release of the joint capsule, sesamoid bones, and short flexor muscles, before using a scalpel to release the plantar phalangeal insertions of the joint capsule and the short flexor muscles. Caution should be exercised, however, as excessive periosteal stripping carries a risk of avascular necrosis to the metatarsal head.[9]

To complement cheilectomy and improve apparent joint motion, a dorsal closing wedge osteotomy of the proximal phalanx[10,11] or the first metatarsal[12] can be added. This procedure improves dorsiflexion but at the expense of plantarflexion; full descriptions of these procedures are described in other articles in this issue.

Results

Among the early reported outcomes of cheilectomy with long-term follow-up, Mann and colleagues[13] reported complete pain relief in 17 of 20 patients at an average follow-up of 68 months. The remaining 3 patients experienced only mild discomfort. Only minimal radiologic progression of arthrosis was noted. Similarly, Mann and Clanton[14] reported 90% considerable or complete resolution of pain among 25 patients undergoing cheilectomy, followed up to 56 months. They also measured range of motion, with 74% of patients experiencing increased range postoperatively, a mean increase of 19°. In a larger series of 93 feet undergoing cheilectomy, and followed up to a mean of 9.6 years, Coughlin and Shurnas[15] noted a 92% success rate in terms of pain relief and function. The mean dorsiflexion improved from 14.5° preoperatively to 38.4° at follow-up. Easley and colleagues[16] recorded the radiographic grade of arthritic degeneration among 68 feet, both preoperatively and at a mean of 63 months after cheilectomy. Most feet showed at least one grade of radiographic worsening by final follow-up, which seems to be of limited significance, given a 90% satisfaction rate, a mean 40-point American Orthopaedic Foot and Ankle Society (AOFAS) hallux rating score improvement and a mean 20° improvement in dorsiflexion following the procedure. A significant incidence of radiographic recurrence of dorsal cheilus was noted, of which only a proportion (9 of 21) were symptomatic.

Radiographic grade does have an association with outcome following cheilectomy. Hattrup and Johnson[3] reported poor outcomes of an unselected group of 58 feet undergoing cheilectomy. Subgroup analysis showed a failure rate of 15% when performed for hallux rigidus with grade I degenerative changes, increasing to 37.5% with established grade III changes. The investigators concluded that cheilectomy is a worthwhile procedure for patients with grade I degeneration, but a joint-sacrificing procedure should be considered when higher grade degeneration is present. Nonetheless, several studies have shown good outcomes.

Data from good-quality comparative trials are lacking. Lau and Daniels[17] reported retrospective data from 24 feet undergoing cheilectomy and 11 feet undergoing interpositional arthroplasty. Cheilectomy yielded superior results in terms of postoperative AOFAS hallux rating scale, great toe strength, and satisfaction. The strength of conclusions were confounded by preoperative radiographic grade, however, with all of the patients in the cheilectomy group showing grade II degenerative appearances, compared with grade III in the interposition arthroplasty group. Similarly, Keiserman and colleagues[18] compared cheilectomy with arthrodesis and interposition arthroplasty, and Pontell and Gudas[19] compared cheilectomy with silastic implant arthroplasty in retrospective trials. Small participant numbers prevented meaningful comparison of results. Beertema and colleagues[20] analyzed results of 28 cheilectomies, 34 arthrodeses, and 28 excision arthroplasties for hallux rigidus. Although they noted significantly better postoperative AOFAS scores in the cheilectomy group, they also noted that the cheilectomy group had a significantly lower average preoperative radiographic grade of disease, again confounding the results.

Feltham and colleagues,[21] in a series of 67 patients undergoing cheilectomy and followed up for a mean of 65 months, noted that patient age influenced outcomes. Patients older than 60 years enjoyed a significantly higher mean postoperative AOFAS score of 89, compared with a mean of 80 for the whole group. Conversely, Mulier and colleagues[22] reported 95% excellent outcomes from cheilectomy performed on 22 feet in 20 young high-level athletes. This selected patient group all had early (grade I or II) radiographic degenerative features, in keeping with Hattrup and Johnson's[3] earlier assertions of radiographic grade as a predictor of outcome following cheilectomy.

Gathering the available data, Roukis[23] performed a systematic review of isolated cheilectomy, identifying data from 706 feet in 23 clinical studies for analysis. The overall rate of requirement for revision surgery was 8.8%. McNeil and colleagues[24] performed a systematic review to assess the quality of evidence for hallux rigidus surgery. Three level III studies were identified,[18–20] all broadly supportive of cheilectomy but not providing good-quality evidence that cheilectomy was better than other operative interventions. Twenty-nine level IV and V studies were analyzed, of which 25 supported cheilectomy as an effective procedure for hallux rigidus.

ARTHROSCOPIC CHEILECTOMY

This procedure is particularly indicated when assessment of the joint is required, for instance, when the radiographic changes are not in keeping with the severity of symptoms and a central osteochondral lesion is suspected (**Fig. 2**). In this case, the best minimally invasive option is arthroscopic, as percutaneous does not allow visualization of the joint other than with fluoroscopy.

Surgical Technique

After spinal or general anesthesia, with the patient supine, the limb is exsanguinated and a thigh tourniquet inflated. While manual traction is applied to the great toe, the MTP joint is distended with 5 mL saline through a dorsomedial injection. Dorsomedial and dorsolateral portals are created using a number 11 blade to create longitudinal incisions through the skin only and using blunt dissection to open the joint capsule. A 2.7-m 30° arthroscope is introduced into the dorsolateral viewing portal, allowing dorsal soft tissue, cheilus and dorsa; metatarsal head to be resected under vision using a 3.5-mm full-radius shaver and a 3.5-mm power abrader through the dorsomedial portal. Resection is continued until 50° to 70° passive dorsiflexion is achieved. Either glue or simple sutures are used to close portals. Postoperative care is the same as described for open cheilectomy.

Technical Variations

Most authors suggest either avoiding joint distraction or just using manual distraction[25–27] to relieve dorsal tissue tension and therefore maximize working space, but Ferkel and colleagues[28] advocate distraction using suspension of the hallux with a

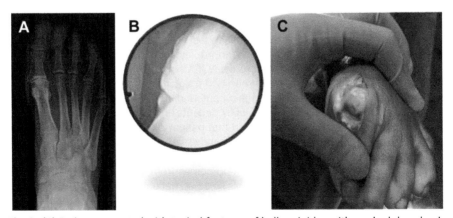

Fig. 2. (A) Patient presented with typical features of hallux rigidus with marked dorsal pain and inability to wear heels, although the radiographs showed very minor changes. Arthroscopy was selected over a percutaneous approach because of this. (B) Arthroscopic photograph of the central cartilage defect. (C) The joint was opened to facilitate debridement and microfracture as there was no significant dorsal degeneration.

sterile Chinese finger trap. The resultant joint distraction may allow greater access to examine the articular surface and even the sesamoid bones. In terms of portals, Ferkel and colleagues recommend a third direct medial portal for fluid inflow, in addition to the standard dorsolateral visualization portal and the dorsomedial instrumentation portal. Lui[29] recommends placement of the dorsolateral and dorsomedial portals further from the EHL tendon than those used for standard arthroscopic examination, to avoid instrument overcrowding in the dorsal work space. A plantarmedial portal is used for evaluation of the central and inferior head and is also useful for instrumentation for microfracture of low-lying cartilage loss or osteochondral lesion.

Finally, some researchers recommend the use of a 1.9-mm-diameter small joint arthroscope, to facilitate access to all parts of the joint. Others use a 2.7-mm-diameter scope, which offers an improved field of view as orientation can be more difficult with a 1.9-mm scope and improved resistance to bending damage. In the senior author's experience, extra-articular shaving with a 4.0-mm scope is superior in both respects and the view that is provided is rewarding. However, this is technically more demanding, particularly in severe osteophytosis. The trocar itself is used as a distractor.

Results

Van Dijk and colleagues[26] reported 2-year follow-up results of arthroscopic debridement for dorsal osteophyte and impinging soft tissues in 12 patients without significant degenerative joint changes (termed the dorsal impingement group) and in 5 patients with hallux rigidus and established arthrosis. Eight (67%) of the dorsal impingement group experienced good or excellent outcomes, compared with only 2 (40%) patients with degenerative hallux rigidus. Iqbal and Chana[27] performed arthroscopic cheilectomy for 15 patients with hallux rigidus and mild to moderate radiographic MTP arthrosis. At a mean follow-up of 9.4 months, 10 patients (67%) experienced complete relief of pain and all patients were either satisfied or very satisfied. The mean time taken to return to normal function was 3.5 weeks. Mean dorsiflexion improved from 7.4° to 47.6°. Ahn and colleagues[30] performed 69 first MTP joint arthroscopies, of which only 3 involved cheilectomy for hallux rigidus. Mean AOFAS hallux rating score improved from 66 to 90 at a mean follow-up of 25 months. One patient was dissatisfied with the procedure because of recurrence of pain, and progression of radiographic arthritic changes was noted.

PERCUTANEOUS CHEILECTOMY
Surgical Technique

Tourniquet is not required for this procedure, and this may even be preferable as the flow of bleeding can help to keep things cooler and carry some bone debris out from the joint. The patient is positioned supine, with the limb free to allow rotation for dorsoplantar (DP) and lateral fluoroscopy. The heel hangs off the end of the table sitting perpendicular to an image intensifier (preferably a mini C-arm to reduce the radiation used), and this gives the best dorsoplantar and lateral joint imaging.

A number 64 Beaver blade is used to make a 4-mm medial longitudinal incision, just dorsal to the first metatarsal neck approximately 1 cm proximal to the osteophyte but remaining plantar to the dorsal digital nerve. The disposable curved elevator is sharp and can be used to create a working space around and proximal to the osteophyte.

Either the 3.1-mm or 4.1-mm Wedge burr can be used depending on the amount of bone resection that is required. The burr is set to high torque but low speed to reduce heat generation; it is also irrigated with saline; however, this only falls on the part of the shaft that is outside. Therefore, it is useful to remove the burr regularly to cool and wash it. Bone debris that collects in the burr significantly increases heat generation, and for these 2 reasons it is important to use the burr in short bursts and remove it to clean and cool it.

The burr is used to abraid the cheilus, until 50° to 70° dosiflexion is achieved. Intraoperative fluoroscopy is used to confirm the extent of resection and is important when learning this technique. The burr is used in a sweeping motion from lateral to medial, gradually working inferiorly increasingly angling the burr. The damage to articular surface of the phalanx is avoided by distracting the toe.

If there is a large dorsal spur, then it is better to undercut it and then shave from below or even just remove the fragments with a mosquito clip (**Fig. 3**). Dorsal osteophyte of the base of the proximal phalanx is addressed in a similar fashion through the same incision, and the toe can be closed down onto the metatarsal head by dorsiflexing it onto the burr. Occasionally, a second lateral longitudinal incision is required to reach the lateral limit of the cheilus, taking care to avoid damage to the abductor hallucis tendon (see **Fig. 3**).

Debris is carefully expressed through the wound, aided by saline irrigation. The joint must be thoroughly cleaned, as bone debris in the joint is a significant irritant and increases the risk of stiffness. Debris within the soft tissues results in delayed wound healing and increases the risk of infection. Thus, the rasp is used to ensure that the soft tissues are cleared. Wounds are sealed with Steri-Strips and dressed. If there is any risk of thermal necrosis, it is better to excise a small ellipse of skin and close. Postoperative care is the same as described for open cheilectomy.

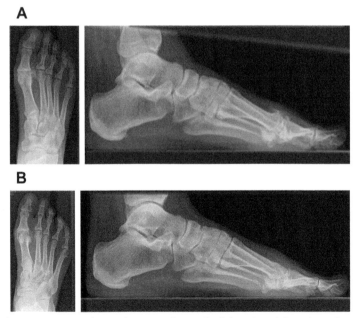

Fig. 3. (*A*) Preoperative radiographs. Note the marked dorsal and dorsolateral osteophytes on the lateral (*i*) and DP (*ii*) views. (*B*) Two-week postoperative radiograph; the dorsal osteophytes have been removed on the lateral view (*i*), with particular focus on the lateral osteophyte on the dorsoplantar view (*ii*).

Results

Little has been published on this technique to date. Morgan and colleagues[31] presented a series of 22 minimally invasive cheilectomy procedures followed up to a median 11 months and a matched comparison group of 25 open cheilectomies followed up to a median of 19 months. Both groups showed significant improvement in Manchester Oxford Foot and Ankle Questionnaire scores. There was a trend toward greater improvement in the open cheilectomy group, although this was not statistically significant. Three patients in the open cheilectomy group required revision to arthrodesis for ongoing pain, compared with none in the minimally invasive group. Small study groups and different lengths of follow-up between the groups limit the strength of conclusions, although minimally invasive cheilectomy seems to be a safe alternative to open surgery. Dawe and colleagues[32] presented results of 16 minimally invasive cheilectomies followed up to 6 months and a comparison group of 22 open cheilectomies followed up to 35 months. Both groups experienced high patient satisfaction, high postoperative AOFAS scores, and similar rates of return to normal footwear and normal function. One superficial wound infection occurred in each group, and 3 revision procedures were required in the open cheilectomy group. Loveday[33] presented results of 29 minimally invasive cheilectomies followed up for a mean of 12 months. Twenty-five (94%) patients were satisfied with the procedure. The 4 patients who were not satisfied were noted to have grade III degenerative joint changes preoperatively. Two patients experienced delayed wound healing, and there was 1 case of transient paresthesia.

Mesa-Ramos and colleagues[34] describe results of percutaneous cheilectomy combined with capsular release and proximal phalanx dorsiflexion osteotomy. Twenty-six cases were followed up for 18 months. Improvements in SF-12 overall health scores, visual analog pain scores, AOFAS scores, and range of motion were observed. There were no infections, although 2 patients (8%) reported ongoing paresthesia 18 months after surgery.

SUMMARY

Cheilectomy is an effective treatment of mild to moderate hallux rigidus. Arthroscopic and fluoroscopy-assisted percutaneous techniques have been developed with the aim of improving patient satisfaction, recovery time, and cosmesis. Early results of these techniques are encouraging, although large, well-designed comparative trials to identify a benefit over open cheilectomy have not yet been conducted.

REFERENCES

1. Beeson P, Phillips C, Corr S, et al. Classification systems for hallux rigidus: a review of the literature. Foot Ankle Int 2008;29:407–14.
2. Thermann H, Becher C. Dorsal cheilectomy, extensive plantar release, and microfracture technique. In: Easley ME, editor. Operative techniques in foot and ankle surgery. Philadelphia: Lippincott Williams and Wilkins; 2011. p. 118–25.
3. Hattrup SJ, Johnson KA. Subjective results of hallux rigidus following treatment with cheilectomy. Clin Orthop Relat Res 1988;226:182–91.
4. Seibert NR, Kadakia AR. Surgical management of hallux rigidus: cheilectomy and osteotomy (phalanx and metatarsal). Foot Ankle Clin N Am 2009;14(1):9–22.
5. Hirose CB, Coughlin MJ, Stevens FR. Arthritis of the foot and ankle. In: Coughlin MJ, Saltzman CL, Anderson RB, editors. Mann's surgery of the foot and ankle, vol. 1. 9th edition. Philadelphia: Elsevier Saunders; 2014. p. 867–1007.

6. Saxena A. The Valenti procedure for hallux limitus/rigidus. J Foot Ankle Surg 2009;34(5):485–8.

7. Grady JF, Axe TM. The modified Valenti procedure for the treatment of hallux limitus. J Foot Ankle Surg 1994;33(4):365–7.

8. Gould JS. Hallux rigidus and arthritis of the first metatarsophalangeal joint. In: Gould JS, editor. The handbook of foot and ankle surgery. An intellectual approach to complex problems. 1st edition. New Delhi (India): Jaypee Brothers Medial Publishers Ltd; 2013. p. 46–55.

9. Brosky TA, Menke CRD, Xenos D. Reconstruction of the first metatarsophalangeal joint following post-cheilectomy avascular necrosis of the first metatarsal head: a case report. J Foot Ankle Surg 2014;48(1):61–9.

10. Kessel L, Bonney G. Hallux rigidus in the adolescent. J Bone Joint Surg Br 1958; 40-B:669–73.

11. Moberg E. A simple operation for hallux rigidus. Clin Orthop Relat Res 1979;(142):55–6.

12. Cavolo DJ, Cavallaro DC, Arrington LE. The Watermann osteotomy for hallux limitus. J Am Podiatry Assoc 1979;69(1):52–7.

13. Mann RA, Coughlin MJ, DuVries HL. Hallux rigidus: a review of the literature and a method of treatment. Clin Orthop Relat Res 1979;142:57–63.

14. Mann RA, Clanton TO. Hallux rigidus: treatment by cheilectomy. J Bone Joint Surg Am 1988;70(3):400–6.

15. Coughlin MJ, Shurnas PS. Hallux rigidus. Grading and long-term results of operative treatment. J Bone Joint Surg Am 2003;85-A(11):2072–88.

16. Easley ME, Davis WH, Anderson RB. Intermediate to long-term follow-up of medial-approach dorsal cheilectomy for hallux rigidus. Foot Ankle Int 1999; 20(3):147–52.

17. Lau JT, Daniels TR. Outcomes following cheilectomy and interpositional arthroplasty in hallux rigidus. Foot Ankle Int 2001;22(6):462–70.

18. Keiserman LS, Sammarco VJ, Sammarco GJ. Surgical treatment of the hallux rigidus. Foot Ankle Clin 2005;10(1):75–96.

19. Pontell D, Gudas CJ. Retrospective analysis of surgical treatment of hallux rigidus/limitus: clinical and radiographic follow-up of hinged, silastic implant arthroplasty and cheilectomy. J Foot Surg 1988;27(6):503–10.

20. Beertema W, Draijer WF, van Os JJ, et al. A retrospective analysis of surgical treatment in patients with symptomatic hallux rigidus: long-term follow-up. J Foot Ankle Surg 2006;45(4):244–51.

21. Feltham GT, Hanks SE, Marcus RE. Age-based outcomes of cheilectomy for the treatment of hallux rigidus. Foot Ankle Int 2001;22(3):192–7.

22. Mulier T, Steenwerckx A, Thienpont E, et al. Results after cheilectomy in athletes with hallux rigidus. Foot Ankle Int 1999;20(4):232–7.

23. Roukis TS. The need for surgical revision after isolated cheilectomy for hallux rigidus: a systematic review. J Foot Ankle Surg 2010;49(5):465–70.

24. McNeil DS, Baumhauer JF, Glazebrook MA. Evidence-based analysis of the efficacy for operative treatment of hallux rigidus. Foot Ankle Int 2013;34(1):15–32.

25. Phisitkul P, Lui TH. Great toe arthroscopy. In: Amendola A, Stone JW, editors. AANA advanced arthroscopy. The foot and ankle. 1st edtion. Philadelphia: Elsevier Saunders; 2010. p. 186–202.

26. van Dijk CN, Veenstra KM, Nuesch BC. Arthroscopic surgery of the metatarsophalangeal first joint. Arthroscopy 1998;14(8):851–5.

27. Iqbal MJ, Chana GS. Arthroscopic cheilectomy for hallux rigidus. Arthroscopy 1998;14(3):307–10.

28. Ferkel RD, Dierckman BD, Phisitkul P. Arthroscopy of the foot and ankle. In: Coughlin MJ, Saltzman CL, Anderson RB, editors. Mann's surgery of the foot and ankle, vol. 2. 9th edition. Philadelphia: Elsevier Saunders; 2014. p. 1723–827.
29. Lui TH. Arthroscopy of the first metatarsophalangeal joint. In: Maffulli N, Easley M, editors. Minimally invasive surgery of the foot and ankle. London: Springer; 2014. p. 57–74.
30. Ahn JH, Choy WS, Lee K-W. Arthroscopy of the first metatarsophalangeal joint in 59 consecutive cases. J Foot Ankle Surg 2012;51(2):161–7.
31. Morgan S, Jones C, Palmer S. Minimally invasive cheilectomy: functional outcome and comparison with open cheilectomy. J Bone 2012;94B(Suppl)XLI:93.
32. Dawe ECJ, Ball T, Annamalai S, et al. Early results of minimally invasive cheilectomy for painful hallux rigidus. J Bone Joint Surg Br 2012;94B(Supp)XXII:33.
33. Loveday D, Guha A, Singh D. Arthritis great toe MTPJ. In: Consensus of the round table. Aspects of orthopaedic foot and ankle surgery. 2nd edition. Paris: 2012. p. 1–9.
34. Mesa-Ramos M, Mesa-Ramos F, Carpintero P. Evaluation of the treatment of hallux rigidus by percutaneous surgery. Acta Orthopaedica Belgica 2008;74: 222–6.

Moberg Osteotomy for Hallux Rigidus

Tibor Warganich, MD[a], Thomas Harris, MD[a,b],*

KEYWORDS

- Moberg osteotomy • Hallux rigidus • Cheilectomy • Proximal phalanx osteotomy
- Hallux limitus

KEY POINTS

- A cheilectomy with Moberg osteotomy is a good option for young and active patients who have failed conservative treatment with moderate and severe hallux rigidus.
- A cheilectomy with Moberg osteotomy has a low complication rate, low revision rate, high patient satisfaction, and can be converted to an arthrodesis should it fail.
- Careful patient counseling, preoperative planning, meticulously placed osteotomies, and stable fixation are critical to optimize outcomes.

INTRODUCTION
Background

Hallux rigidus is a degenerative osteoarthritis of the first metatarsophalangeal (MTP) joint. It is marked by pain and a decrease in the arc of motion of the first MTP joint. It is sometimes also referred to as hallux flexus, hallux limitus, metatarsus elevatus, or dorsal bunion,[1,2] and was originally described by Davies-Colley[3] in 1887. Typically patients have more pronounced pain with dorsiflexion relative to plantarflexion, presumably caused by impingement on a degenerative dorsal osseous rim. The loss of functional range of motion mostly with dorsiflexion is caused by this osteophyte formation on the dorsal surface of the first proximal phalanx base and first metatarsal (MT) head.[3–5] Patients commonly report pain at the first MTP joint with prolonged activity; however, as the disease progresses patients complain of pain at rest. It is estimated to affect 3% of adults more than 50 years of age and is second only to hallux valgus with regard to great toe orthopedic disorders.[6] The predominant loss of dorsiflexion and the pain with terminal dorsiflexion is the rational behind the dorsal closing

Disclosure: The authors have nothing to disclose.
[a] Department of Orthopaedics, Harbor-UCLA, 1000 West Carson Street, #422, Torrance, CA 90502, USA; [b] Congress Medical Associates, Foot and Ankle Surgery, Harbor-UCLA, 800 South Raymond Avenue, Second Floor, Pasadena, CA 91105, USA
* Corresponding author. Congress Medical Associates, Foot and Ankle Surgery, Harbor-UCLA, 800 South Raymond Avenue, Second Floor, Pasadena, CA 91105.
E-mail address: thomasgharrismd@gmail.com

Foot Ankle Clin N Am 20 (2015) 433–450
http://dx.doi.org/10.1016/j.fcl.2015.04.006
1083-7515/15/$ – see front matter © 2015 Elsevier Inc. All rights reserved.

foot.theclinics.com

wedge osteotomy. Bonney and Macnab[7] initially described the proximal phalanx dorsal closing wedge osteotomy in 1952 for patients less than 18 years old. However, in 1979 Moberg,[8] to whom the procedure is sometimes attributed, popularized the procedure by extending the indications to include active adults.[8] The dorsal closing wedge osteotomy steals motion from plantarflexion and passes it to dorsiflexion, thereby shifting the first MTP's less painful arc of motion (plantarflexion) into the more physiologic arc of motion (dorsiflexion), thus mitigating the pain associated with the extremes of first MTP extension.[8] More recently, favorable results and patient satisfaction scores have expanded the indication to include active adults with more severe grades of the disease.[8–12]

Several surgical treatment options exist for hallux rigidus and careful consideration must be given to the patient, level of disease, and the performing surgeon's experience. The Moberg osteotomy is rarely used as a sole procedure but is routinely used to augment the cheilectomy.[11] It was not until 1993 that Desai and colleagues[13] described combining the Moberg osteotomy with the cheilectomy. Five years later, Blyth and colleagues[14] were the first to publish a peer-reviewed article on combining the two procedures. Since that time the combination of the two procedures has become widespread and popular among surgeons. Several investigators have reported favorable results, improved American Orthopaedic Foot and Ankle Society (AOFAS) scores, and patient satisfaction with the Moberg osteotomy combined with a cheilectomy. Performing a Moberg osteotomy together with a cheilectomy adds little additional surgical time, exposure, or dissection, and still affords the option of more aggressive future revisions should the surgery fail.[15]

Pathophysiology and Cause

The primary cause of hallux rigidus is still widely debated and not completely understood, but many speculations exist. There have been few studies that have shown a causality to hallux rigidus and thus, although the corrective surgery is common and widely accepted, the pathologic derangement has yet to be clinically and definitively proved.[16] Among the likely causative factors that have been proposed are trauma,[17–19] improper shoe wear,[3,20] genetic traits, excessively long first MT,[18,21] a hypermobile first MT,[18] immobility of the first ray,[18,22] osteochondritis dissecans (OCD) (particularly in the adolescent population[5,17,23]), altered center of rotation of first MTP joint (center of rotation outside the MT head[24,25]), a pronated foot,[21,26] and the summation of microtrauma leading to degeneration.[27] In addition to primary causes of hallux rigidus, there are several secondary causes from inflammatory systemic conditions that can lead to disease (gout, rheumatoid arthritis, and seronegative arthritis[28]).

History and Clinical Findings

Hallux rigidus is most common in adults (particularly women), is often bilateral, and increases from roughly 3% at age 50 years[6] to almost 50% after age 65 years.[29] Patients typically complain of dull, activity-related pain in the first MTP joint, particularly with push-off during gait.[28] Patients may complain of pain with high-heeled shoes, flexible shoe wear,[28] walking uphill, or any activity that increases the first MTP dorsiflexion and thus the painful impingement on dorsal osteophytes. In more advanced disease, the dorsal osteophytes can be bulky and patients may also complain of trouble fitting shoes or irritation over the first MTP head as the dorsal osteophyte causes mechanical obstruction and inflammation to the overlaying joint capsule, synovium, and soft tissues.[28] Patients often have pain at rest, and may be better suited for an MTP arthrodesis rather than a joint preserving procedure.

On examination there is typically decreased dorsiflexion with almost normal plantar-flexion. Although both extremes in motion can be painful, plantarflexion is often more painful in advanced disease, which is thought to be caused by compression of the inflamed dorsal capsule against the osteophyte.[28] Often the first MTP joint is enlarged, erythematous, and swollen, with a possible Tinel on the medial dorsal cutaneous nerve from compression by the osteophyte.[28] Although the arthritic changes of hallux rigidus progress with increasing age, they are not necessarily correlated with symptoms.[30] These patients often do well with a cheilectomy alone because they experience little pain with range of motion.[31] For patients with moderate to severe disease, it can be useful to perform a grind test, in which the clinician provides an axial load while rotating of the MTP joint to elicit pain. Patients who have pain with the MTP joint in neutral or plantar flexion often have more extensive disease and may not be ideal candidates for the cheilectomy and Moberg osteotomy. However, they may also have an osteochondral lesion that elicits pain with grinding, and not extensive arthritic disease, so the authors do not routinely perform a grind test given the confusion it can cause.

Diagnostic Studies and Staging

Three weight-bearing plain radiographs (anteroposterior [AP], lateral, oblique) are typically all that is needed to diagnose and shape a treatment plan for hallux rigidus.[28] Standing radiographs are essential to accurately gauge the amount of joint space narrowing and prevent the phalanges from extending and obscuring the amount of dorsal osteophytes.[31] The AP view is useful in showing medial and lateral osteophytes, sclerotic changes, and subchondral cysts.[28] The amount of disease can be overestimated in the AP view if the dorsal osteophytes on the phalanges overlie the joint space.[2,28] The lateral view is often the most informative and shows the extent of the dorsal osteophytes, status of the joint space, possible loose bodies, and early disease with degenerative changes seen only at the dorsal surface of the joint.[2] The oblique view can be useful in more advanced disease because it shows arthritic changes of the plantar surface of the joint.[28] Advanced imaging can be useful if osteochondral defects are suspected. MRI may be indicated in cases of trauma, normal radiographs, young patients, or when there is suspected chondral damage, loose body, or a developing OCD lesion. Computed tomography (CT) can be helpful in cases of bony defects, advanced OCD lesions with free fragments, or if suspecting metatarsosesamoid joint arthritis. If metatarsosesamoid arthritis is present and severe, a Moberg osteotomy and cheilectomy may not address all the patient's symptoms.

Many grading systems have been suggested but there is no gold standard. One system was proposed by Hattrup and Johnson[32] in 1988 and is used to help guide treatment. Hattrup and Johnson[32] categorized hallux rigidus into 3 grades based solely on plain radiographs. Grade I disease is a painful first MTP joint with mild osteophytes and normal joint space. Grade II disease is marked by joint space narrowing, sclerosis, and moderate dorsal osteophytes. Grade III disease is characterized by absence of first MTP joint space and severe osteophyte formation.[32] In 2003, Coughlin and Shurnas[33] described a more comprehensive grading system that is now widely accepted. Their classification system categorized hallux rigidus into 5 grades depending on both the clinical examination and radiographic findings. Grade 0 disease is a painless, stiff joint with normal radiographs and 10% to 20% loss of range of motion. Grade I disease is a mildly painful joint at the extremes of motion with radiographs showing a small dorsal osteophyte plus minimal joint space narrowing and 20% to 50% loss of range of motion. Grade II disease is a more constant, moderately painful joint with radiographs showing a moderate dorsal osteophyte plus mild to moderate joint space narrowing with 50% to 75% loss of range of motion. Patients with grade III disease have pain that is mostly constant but spared at midrange, 75% to 100% loss of range of motion, and radiographs with severe osteophytes and substantial joint space narrowing. Grade IV disease is marked by severe stiffness and pain throughout the range of motion (including the midrange) and radiographs with severe dorsal osteophytes and substantial joint space narrowing.[33]

Conservative Treatment

For patients with mild symptoms and occasional complaints, hallux rigidus is treated well conservatively. The first line of treatment consists of nonsteroidal antiinflammatory medications, corticosteroids, rest, ice, and activity modification, which is intended to decrease the amount of dorsiflexion of the first MTP and decrease mechanical pressure on the dorsal osteophytes. Limiting the amount of painful dorsiflexion can be achieved by wearing stiffer shoes, using an orthotic insert that has a rigid extension under the first MTP joint (Morton extension), or choosing exercises that limit motion at the first MTP joint (eg, swimming and cycling). Avoiding high-heeled shoes and choosing shoe wear with high toe-box limits painful pressure on dorsal osteophytes. Compliance varies with individual patients and may not be effective for advanced disease. However, Smith and colleagues[30] reported that pain remained the same in 22 out of 24 feet in a follow-up study of patients treated nonoperatively at an average of 14 years.

INDICATIONS/CONTRAINDICATIONS
Indications

Although Bonney and Macnab[7] initially described the procedure for adolescents in 1952, Moberg[8] in 1979 extended the indications to include adults who were active. The Moberg osteotomy is generally reserved for moderate to severe hallux rigidus (Hattrup and Johnson grades II to III)[10] that has failed conservative treatment. The Moberg osteotomy has been used as a stand-alone procedure with good results, but is typically used to augment the cheilectomy in recent surgical trends.[9,13,14] Patients should also show limited dorsiflexion and normal plantarflexion of the MTP joint so that there is enough range of motion to steal from the plantarflexion and a deficit dorsally to justify shifting the functional range of motion. Young, active patients with moderate disease and preserved plantarflexion are the ideal surgical candidates (**Table 1**).

Contraindications

It is imperative to perform a detailed physical examination and radiographic work-up. Patients with normal passive dorsiflexion are unlikely to improve dramatically with increasing the dorsiflexion. Likewise if there is no passive plantarflexion to steal from, the osteotomy is contraindicated because a significant shift in functional range

Table 1	
Indications and contraindications	
Indications	**Contraindications**
Young or active adults	Normal passive dorsiflexion
Moderate to severe hallux rigidus (Hattrup and Johnson grades II and III)	No passive plantarflexion
	End-stage degenerative changes with bone-on-bone arthritis
Used to augment cheilectomy	Older, less active patients
Limited dorsiflexion and normal plantarflexion	

of motion cannot occur.[28] In addition, patients with end-stage degenerative changes and loss of cartilage below the dorsal surface may have unfavorable outcomes[2] and persistent pain because Moberg osteotomy is designed to decompress the dorsal joint pressures. Therefore older, less active patients with global bone-on-bone degeneration with little MTP joint motion do not have as favorable outcomes and may benefit more from an arthrodesis (see **Table 1**).

SURGICAL TECHNIQUE
Preoperative Planning

- Three weight-bearing views of the foot (in non–weight-bearing views, the toes are in extension and the proximal phalanx can obscure dorsal osteophytes on the MT).
- Special attention is paid to the lateral view because this gives an appreciation of the extent of dorsal osteophytes and the amount of joint space narrowing (**Fig. 1**).
- An AP radiograph can overestimate the amount of joint destruction.
- If chondral injury or OCD is suspected, consider MRI or CT.
- Record preoperative passive range of motion (plantarflexion and dorsiflexion) and postoperative improvement in functional arc of motion.
- Counsel the patient on the risks and benefits of the procedure, including the trade-off of sacrificing normal plantarflexion for the more functional dorsiflexion (**Box 1**).

Prep and Patient Positioning

- Patient is positioned supine with a bump under the hip to bring the foot into neutral rotation if necessary.
- A tourniquet is applied to the thigh if the patient's passive range of motion is to be tested intraoperatively without tethering of the long flexor or extensor tendons. In addition, ankle tourniquets can be used in awake patients because these are less painful than tourniquets on the thigh.

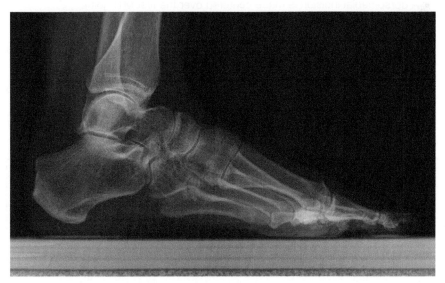

Fig. 1. Preoperative lateral radiograph showing grade II hallux rigidus with joint space narrowing and a dorsal osteophyte on the first MT head.

Box 1
Preoperative planning

- Three weight-bearing radiographs
- Lateral view yields most information on joint destruction
- MRI or CT if OCD is suspected
- Record preoperative passive range of motion
- Counsel patient on loss of plantarflexion for gain in dorsiflexion and possible arthrodesis if there is bone-on-bone arthritis found intraoperatively

---

- The procedure is performed under an ankle block with intravenous sedation or laryngeal mask airway (LMA).
- Preoperative antibiotics are given within 30 minutes of incision as per protocol.
- Intraoperative fluoroscopy should be available (**Box 2**).

Surgical Approach

- A dorsomedial incision is made just medial to the extensor hallucis longus (EHL) (**Fig. 2**).
- Hash marks are recommended to aid in skin approximation at closure.
- EHL is retracted laterally and the dorsomedial nerve is retracted medially.
- Alternatively, a directly medial incision can be made.
- A medial incision may limit adequate exposure of lateral joint line.
- A previous medial incision does not preclude a dorsomedial incision since it is safe, but extra care should be taken to avoid overzealous retraction or soft tissue dissection.

Surgical Procedure

Part 1: cheilectomy

- A dorsomedial incision is made centered over the first MTP joint.
- Carefully dissect, identify, and protect the EHL and dorsomedial nerve.
- Retract EHL laterally and dorsomedial nerve medially.
- Expose the MTP joint capsule and perform an arthrotomy in line with the skin incision.
  - Tag the capsule with 2-0 Vicryl sutures for later closure.
- Two Senn retractors move the soft tissue medial and lateral, bringing the full MTP joint into view (**Fig. 3**).
- Plantarflex the MTP joint to expose the joint surface.
  - Note the extent and nature of chondral defect.

Box 2
Preparation and patient positioning

- Supine with a bump under ipsilateral hip to bring foot into neutral position
- Thigh tourniquet
- Ankle block with LMA or intravenous sedation versus ETGA (endotracheal general anesthesia)
- Antibiotics 30 minutes before incision
- Intraoperative fluoroscopy

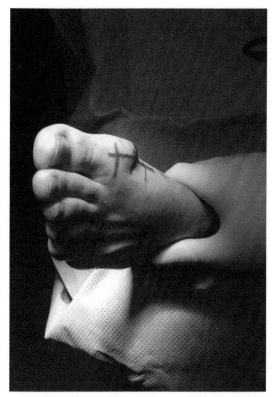

Fig. 2. The placement of a dorsomedial incision medial to the EHL over the dorsal osteophyte.

- ■ Consider arthrodesis if there are extensive, eburnated cartilage defects.
- Remove 1 to 2 mm of medial osteophyte from the MT head with a reciprocating saw.
- Perform the cheilectomy of the MT head with a reciprocating saw.
- Resect the osteophyte and part of the MT head with the cartilage defect. Up to 30% of the MT head can be resected without destabilizing the joint.
- Osteotomy should be flush with dorsal surface of the MT neck.
- A dorsal osteophyte of the proximal phalanx can be removed in a similar manner or with a rongeur.
- Inspect the lateral side of the MTP joint and remove osteophytes with a rongeur or narrow osteotome.
  - ○ Often these osteophytes are not appreciated on plain films.
- Cuts are cooled with irrigation.

Part 2: Moberg osteotomy

- Expose the proximal phalanx enough to protect the flexor hallucis longus (FHL) with an instrument during the osteotomy if necessary.
- Under the guidance of fluoroscopy, place a 1.57-mm (0.062-inch) Kirschner wire from medial to lateral as close as possible to the joint surface to guide the osteotomy cut (**Fig. 4**).

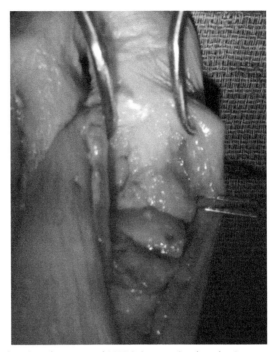

Fig. 3. A cadaver showing the exposed MTP joint proximal to the Senn retractors. The EHL is retracted laterally and the dorsomedial nerve medially.

- ○ Use fluoroscopy to ensure that the Kirschner wire is extra-articular.
- ○ The osteotomy cut should be close to the joint surface to maximize the gains in dorsiflexion, but not so close that it causes a fracture of the proximal fragment or prevents there being enough bone stock for fixation.

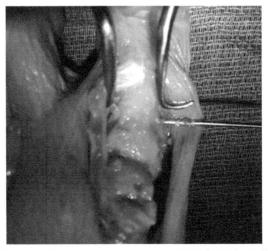

Fig. 4. A cadaver showing a Kirschner wire placed medial to lateral parallel to the joint surface to guide the proximal osteotomy.

- The first cut is made with an oscillating 0.5-cm blade distal to the Kirschner wire guide and parallel to the joint. Cool the osteotomy with irrigation.
  - Protect the EHL with retractors from possible laceration resulting from friction from the side of the saw blade.
    - If the EHL is lacerated, it should be repaired acutely and postoperative rehabilitation adjusted accordingly.
  - The osteotomy is stopped before perforation of the plantar cortex.
    - This is done for 2 reasons: (1) it helps prevent iatrogenic laceration of the FHL, and (2) it maintains bony stability of the phalanx for the second cut.
- The second cut is made 2 to 4 mm distal to the first cut and is angled to converge with the first cut at the plantar cortex to complete the wedge resection.
  - The authors recommend using a sterile ruler to mark out the second osteotomy.
  - Monitoring the dorsal cortex is an easy and reliable way to ensure parallel cuts.
  - It is critical that the osteotomy cuts are parallel to one another or a varus/valgus deformity will ensue.
    - However, mild angular cuts can be made intentionally if desired to correct for preoperative hallux valgus or hallux varus.
  - As with the first cut, the osteotomy is stopped short of penetrating the plantar cortex to prevent injury to the FHL.
- The plantar cortex is then weakened with successive holes made by a 1.57-mm (0.062-inch) Kirschner wire and then greensticked to finish the cut.
- Manual dorsiflexion reduces the fracture and confirms the accuracy of the cuts.
- As for all cuts, cooling irrigation helps prevent thermal damage and possible delayed union or nonunion (**Fig. 5**).

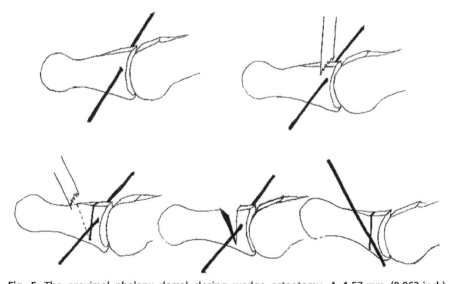

Fig. 5. The proximal phalanx dorsal closing wedge osteotomy. A 1.57-mm (0.062-inch) Kirschner wire is inserted medial to lateral under fluoroscopy to be close and parallel to the joint. The first cut is made parallel and distal to the guiding Kirschner wire and stopped short of the plantar cortex. The second cut is made 2 to 4 mm distal to the first cut and aimed obliquely to converge with the first cut on the plantar cortex. The wedge of bone is resected and the osteotomy is reduced with manual pressure and held with a provisional Kirschner wire.

Part 3: fixation

- Multiple options have been described for fixation of the osteotomy site, including minifragment plate and screws, percutaneous Kirschner wires (usually 1.37 mm [0.054 inch]), staples, partially threaded lag screws, 28-G cerclage wires, or a Plaple (a combination of a staple and a plate made by Arthrex, Naples, FL). The author's preferred method of fixation is the Plaple; however, excellent results have been seen with both the 28-G wire and percutaneous Kirschner wires. Previously, 28-G wire through two 45° holes exiting dorsomedially has been used, which was twisted to maintain tension. Although the fixation is cost-effective and low profile, there are concerns of wire cutout and stability. Kirschner wires placed percutaneously across the fracture site were also used, but they carry a risk of infection, can be unsightly, and are slightly painful when removed.
- The Plaple minimizes the chance of proximal fragment fracture, is low profile, avoids possible infection compared with percutaneous Kirschner wires, and provides mild compression across the fracture.
- The Plaple is oriented with the staple end inserted into the subchondral bone of the proximal fragment and the screw end through the distal fragment, thus providing compression.
- Measure the ideal length of the plate with a sterile ruler (**Fig. 6**).
- Using a 1.57-mm (0.062-inch) Kirschner wire, predrill a pilot hole for the blade in the proximal fragment, which is well centered and in subchondral bone.
- Be mindful when predrilling the pilot hole that the proximal phalanx is concave, and do not place the proximal end of the Plaple into the joint accidentally.
- The assistant then dorsiflexes the toe, reduces the fracture, and provides preliminary compression across the osteotomy.

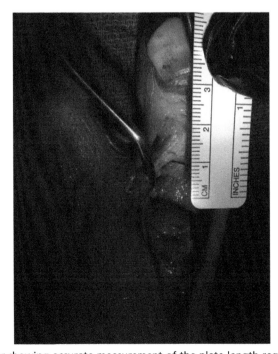

Fig. 6. A cadaver showing accurate measurement of the plate length required.

- o Alternatively, the osteotomy can be reduced and held with a Kirschner wire (**Fig. 7**).
- Using the appropriate length Plaple as a template, the screw site is then marked and predrilled with a 1.7-mm drill through the dorsal cortex only.
- The blade end of the Plaple is then inserted into the pilot hole of the proximal fragment.
  - o A tamp can be used to ensure the Plaple is flush with the bone.
- The 1.7-mm drill then revisits the screw hole and makes it bicortical.
- The screw length is measured with a depth gauge and the screw is advanced in the distal fragment, providing compression and stability (**Figs. 8–10**).
  - o It is helpful if an assistant maintains and provides compression while the screw is advanced.
- Nearby cancellous bone graft from the osteotomy slice can be morcellized and used over the osteotomy site.
- The proximal phalanx is then examined for angular alignment and put through a gentle range of motion to access for stability.
- The wound is then irrigated.
- The arthrotomy is closed using previously placed 2-0 Vicryl to easily find the capsule.
- Deep capsule is closed with interrupted, nonabsorbable 2-0 suture.
- The tourniquet is released and stable hemostasis is obtained with electrocautery.
- As much soft tissue as possible is reapproximated over the wound using 2-0 Vicryl.
- The skin is closed with 4-0 nylon in a simple interrupted fashion.
- The incision is covered with a nonadherent dressing, gauze, soft padding, compressive dressing, and then a hard-soled postoperative shoe.

COMPLICATIONS AND MANAGEMENT

- Soft tissue injury leading to laceration of EHL, FHL, or dorsomedial cutaneous nerve.[14] To avoid injury to FHL, consider making incomplete osteotomies with the saw blade and finishing the plantar cut with a series of drill holes. To limit injury to the EHL, avoid placing the tendon under unnecessary tension with excessive plantarflexion of the MTP joint.

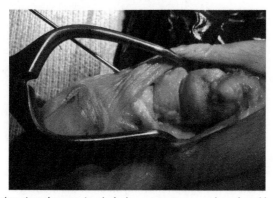

Fig. 7. A cadaver showing the proximal phalanx osteotomy reduced and held in place with a Kirschner wire.

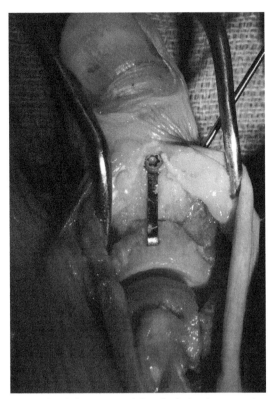

Fig. 8. A cadaver showing final placement of the Plaple (Arthrex, Naples, FL) with the blade in the proximal fragment, screw in the distal fragment, and the fracture well reduced.

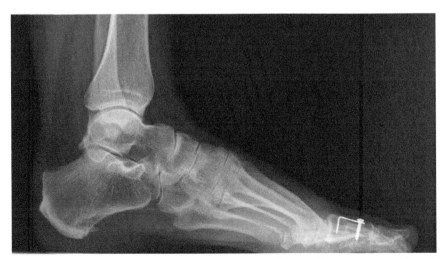

Fig. 9. Postoperative lateral radiograph showing union of the Moberg osteotomy. Note the removal of the dorsal MT head osteophyte and increased dorsal angulation of the proximal phalanx.

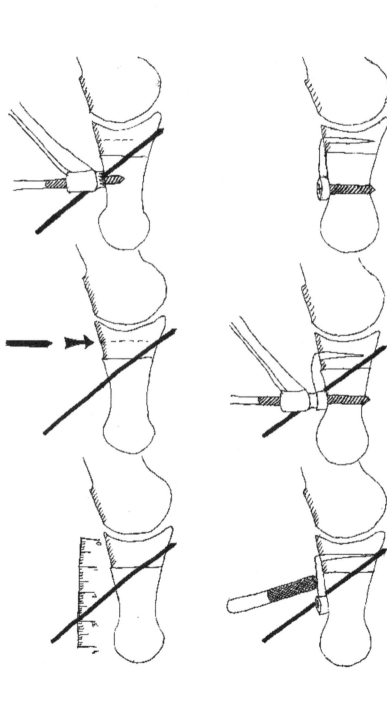

Fig. 10. The author's preferred method of fixation of the proximal phalanx osteotomy using a Plaple (Arthrex, Naples, FL). A Kirschner wire holds the reduction preliminarily and the optimal length is measured with a ruler. The proximal fragment is predrilled with a Kirschner wire centered in the subchondral bone. Using the appropriate length Plaple, the screw site is marked and predrilled through the dorsal cortex only. The Plaple is then oriented with the blade proximally and advanced into the pilot hole and tamped flush with the bone. The distal screw hole is revisited and made bicortical. The screw is advanced through the eyelet of the Plaple while maintaining reduction and achieving compression with bicortical fixation.

- Intra-articular extension from the osteotomy. Consider placing 1.57-mm (0.062-inch) Kirschner wires mirroring the joint line medial to lateral under fluoroscopy to guide the proximal osteotomy.
- Varus/valgus deformity from osteotomy.[9] This pitfall is typically caused by inadequate soft tissue exposure and failing to place the cuts parallel to the direction of the joint line. Using a sterile ruler can aid in making the second osteotomy parallel to the first.
- Comminution of the proximal fragment from an osteotomy placed too close to the joint. Place the drill hole for the tension wire as close to the joint as possible. If using cerclage wire, tension the wire from proximal to distal, especially when first performing the osteotomy.
- Nonunion.[34] This risk is rare if there is good compression, stable fixation across fracture site, and thermal damage is minimized with irrigation.
- Malunion.[34]
- Osteoarthritis of the interphalangeal joint.[34,35]
- Infection.[10,36]
- Symptomatic hardware (prevalence is about 5%[10,36]). If there is persistent pain over prominent hardware, it can be removed through the previous incision.
- Arthrofibrosis requiring MUA (manipulation under anesthesia).[10]
- Secondary metatarsalgia.[10,14,35]
- Persistent pain or recurrent pain.[13,35–37]
- Persistent symptoms requiring revision surgery or arthrodesis.[9,13,14,35,36,38] Careful preoperative evaluation is critical to detect patients with end-stage arthritis or little range of motion, who are more successfully treated with arthrodesis (**Box 3**).

POSTOPERATIVE CARE

- Hard-soled shoes for 3 to 6 weeks postoperatively.
- Weight bearing as tolerated on the heel on postoperative day 1, and then weight bearing as tolerated on plantigrade foot after the first postoperative visit.
- Follow-up in clinic for a wound check in 7 to 10 days postoperatively.

Box 3
Complications

- Iatrogenic soft tissue laceration (EHL, FHL, dorsomedial cutaneous nerve)
- Proximal phalanx osteotomy extending into joint
- Varus or valgus deformity
- Comminution of proximal bone fragment
- Nonunion
- Malunion
- Osteoarthritis of interphalangeal joint
- Infection
- Symptomatic hardware
- Arthrofibrosis
- Secondary metatarsalgia
- Persistent pain
- Recurrent pain requiring revision or arthrodesis

- Patients are encouraged to massage the wound once it is healed to decrease adhesions and chances of complex regional pain syndrome.
- Dorsiflexion with passive range-of-motion exercises start at postoperative week 1 or 2, depending on stability of fixation.
- Plantarflexion with passive range-of-motion exercises should start at postoperative week 4 to avoid overdistraction of the osteotomy site (if the great toe's resting posture is in extension with weight bearing, more aggressive passive range of motion with plantarflexion is encouraged).
- Elevate the extremity strictly for 2 to 3 days postoperatively and whenever possible after that.

OUTCOMES

The current literature suggests that a Moberg osteotomy combined with a cheilectomy is usually successful and well received in patients with painful hallux rigidus who have failed conservative treatment.[15] However, there is a paucity of high-level evidence in most of these studies.[15] It is generally recommended for mild or advanced disease[10] in patients who are active and would not tolerate an arthrodesis. The rationale behind the Moberg osteotomy is to decompress the MTP joint and decrease contact pressures between the dorsal aspect of the base of the proximal phalanx and the dorsal surface of the MTP head. This decompression is accomplished, as Moberg[8] described, by converting plantar flexion to dorsiflexion. The osteotomy shifts the nonpainful arc of motion from plantarflexion to the more functional position of dorsiflexion.

Citron and Neil[34] reported their long-term follow-up results with Moberg osteotomy as a stand-alone procedure for hallux rigidus on 10 toes of 8 patients. At an average follow-up of 22 years, only 1 toe required revision surgery (conversion to arthrodesis), all toes were pain free initially and 5 toes remained pain free at follow-up, and 4 toes had pain but it did not restrict walking.[34] Blyth and colleagues[14] in 1998 were the first to report peer-reviewed outcomes on 14 feet with an average follow-up of 4 years with grade I, II, and III disease. Most patients had improved pain (83%) with good or excellent outcomes (77%) and only 1 patient went on to arthrodesis. Thomas and Smith[9] showed in a retrospective study of 24 feet over an average of 5 years that 96% of patients would have the procedure done again and there were no reported complications. Kilmartin[35] showed in a prospective study that 89% of patients were satisfied with the procedure, 8% required hardware removal, and there was an average improvement of 45 points in the AOFAS metatarsophalangeal joint–interphalangeal joint scale. In a retrospective study with 47 feet, Wingenfeld and colleagues[38] showed that 77% would do surgery again, 82% were satisfied with the surgery, and there was 1 case requiring revision. O'Malley and colleagues[10] reported results in severe hallux rigidus (grade III disease) on 81 feet with an average follow-up of 4 years with 85% of patients satisfied with the procedure, 4 patients requiring eventual arthrodesis, 3 patients requiring hardware removal, and no nonunions or malunions.

Overall, the results of a recent meta-analysis of 11 studies over 17 years on 374 toes undergoing Moberg osteotomy with cheilectomy showed that the need for revision is low (4.8%), patient satisfaction is high (77%), pain was eliminated or improved in 89%, and the AOFAS metatarsophalangeal–interphalangeal scoring scale improved an average of 39 points.[15]

SUMMARY

Hallux rigidus is a common condition causing pain at the first MTP joint in roughly 1 in 40 adults more than the age of 50 years and occasionally in adolescents.[6] Historically, cheilectomy has been performed for mild disease with favorable results.[1,28] In 2004, Coughlin and Shurnas[39] retrospectively studied 110 toes undergoing a cheilectomy alone with an average follow-up of 9.6 years and reported significant improvements in dorsiflexion, AOFAS scores, pain, and function (92% of patients).[39] For mild to moderate disease, other investigators have reported results with a combined Moberg osteotomy and cheilectomy and showed that most patients had significant improvement in pain and function.[9,13–15,35–38] Previously, advanced hallux rigidus with widespread articular degeneration was an indication for arthrodesis.[39] However, many surgeons have pushed the indication of cheilectomy with Moberg osteotomy to include more advanced disease with success.[10,11]

Careful preoperative patient evaluation and work-up are important to define the select subpopulation of individuals who will benefit the most from the combined procedure. The ideal patient is has dorsal osteophytes, normal plantar flexion and limited dorsiflexion, with at least some pain-free range of motion, and is young or active. It is also a beneficial adjunct for patients who want to wear high-heeled shoes, given the added dorsiflexion it provides. It is important to counsel patients with advanced articular degeneration (>50%) and a painful arc of motion that this procedure may not alleviate all of their symptoms and there is a chance (roughly 5%)[10] of a need for an arthrodesis. During the procedure, there are many internal fixation methods available, all with their own sets of advantages and disadvantages. To our knowledge, the literature does not clearly support one fixation method rather than another. We prefer to use the Plaple, because it provides some compression across the osteotomy, is stable, and is low profile in the proximal fragment and under the skin. Overall, patients do well with the combined procedure with a high satisfaction rate, significant pain relief, improved AOFAS scores, an increase in the functional arc of motion, and low complication and revision rates.

REFERENCES

1. Mann RA, Clanton TO. Hallux rigidus: treatment by cheilectomy. J Bone Joint Surg Am 1988;70:400–6.
2. Shereff MJ, Baumhauer JF. Hallux rigidus and osteoarthrosis of the first metatarsophalangeal joint. J Bone Joint Surg Am 1998;80:898–908.
3. Davies-Colley M. Contraction of the metatarsophalangeal joint of the great toe. Br Med J 1887;1:728–34.
4. DuVries HV. Surgery of the foot. St Louis (MO): Mosby Year Book; 1959. p. 392–9, 7.
5. Goodfellow J. Aetiology of hallux rigidus. Proc R Soc Med 1966;59:821–4.
6. Gould N, Schneider W, Ashikaga T. Epidemiological survey of foot problems in the continental United States: 1978-1979. Foot Ankle 1980;1:8–10.
7. Bonney G, Macnab I. Hallux valgus and hallux rigidus; a critical survey of operative results. J Bone Joint Surg Br 1952;34-B:366–85.
8. Moberg E. A simple operation for hallux rigidus. Clin Orthop Relat Res 1979;(142):55–6.
9. Thomas PJ, Smith RW. Proximal phalanx osteotomy for the surgical treatment of hallux rigidus. Foot Ankle Int 1999;20:3–12.
10. O'Malley MJ, Basran HS, Gu Y, et al. Treatment of advanced stages of hallux rigidus with cheilectomy and phalangeal osteotomy. J Bone Joint Surg Am 2013;95:606–10.
11. Harris TG. Moberg osteotomy - dorsiflexion osteotomy of the proximal phalanx. OrthopaedicsOne Articles. In: OrthopaedicsOne - the orthopaedic knowledge network. Available at: http://www.orthopaedicsone.com/x/dQYCAg. Created Jun 03, 2010 21:17. Accessed July 25, 2012. 04:15 ver.15.

12. Parvizi J, Kitaoka HB. Proximal phalangeal (Moberg) osteotomy. Master techniques in orthopaedic surgery. 3rd edition. Foot Ankle; 2002. p. 39–54.
13. Desai VV, Zafiropoulos G, Dias JJ, et al. Hallux rigidus: a case against joint destruction. Presented at the British Orthopaedic Foot Surgery Society Meeting, 12 November 1993. J Bone Joint Surg Br 1994;76(Suppl 2, 3):95.
14. Blyth MJ, Mackay DC, Kinninmonth AW. Dorsal wedge osteotomy in the treatment of hallux rigidus. J Foot Ankle Surg 1998;37:8–10.
15. Roukis TS. Outcomes after cheilectomy with phalangeal dorsiflexory osteotomy for hallux rigidus: a systematic review. J Foot Ankle Surg 2010;49:479–87.
16. Botek G, Anderson MA. Etiology, pathophysiology, and staging of hallux rigidus. Clin Podiatr Med Surg 2011;28:229–43, vii.
17. McMaster MJ. The pathogenesis of hallux rigidus. J Bone Joint Surg Br 1978;60: 82–7.
18. Root ML, Orien WP, Weed JH. Motion at specific joints of the foot. In: Root SA, editor. Normal and abnormal function of the foot. 1st edition. Los Angeles (CA): Clinical Biomechanics Corporation; 1977. p. 46–60, 350–70.
19. Coughlin MJ, Shurnas PS. Hallux rigidus: demographics, etiology, and radiographic assessment. Foot Ankle Int 2003;24:731–43.
20. McMurray TP. Treatment of hallux valgus and rigidus. Br Med J 1936;2:218–21.
21. Nilsonne H. Hallux rigidus and its treatment. Acta Orthop Scand 1930;1:295–303.
22. Chang TJ, Camasta CA. Hallux limitus and hallux rigidus. In: Banks AS, McGlamry ED, editors. McGlamry's comprehensive textbook of foot and ankle surgery. 3rd edition. Philadelphia: Lippincott Williams & Wilkins; 2001. p. 679–711.
23. Kessel L, Bonney G. Hallux rigidus in the adolescent. J Bone Joint Surg Br 1958; 40-B:669–73.
24. Sammarco GJ. Biomechanics of the foot. In: Frankel VH, Nordin M, editors. Basic biomechanics of the skeleton system. Philadelphia: Lea & Febiger; 1980. p. 193–219.
25. Shereff MJ, Bejjani FJ, Kummer FJ. Kinematics of the first metatarsophalangeal joint. J Bone Joint Surg Am 1986;68:392–8.
26. Bingold AC, Collins DH. Hallux rigidus. J Bone Joint Surg Br 1950;32-B:214–22.
27. Giannestras NJ. Foot disorders: medical and surgical management. 2nd edition. Philadelphia: Lea & Febiger; 1973. p. 400.
28. Keiserman LS, Sammarco VJ, Sammarco GJ. Surgical treatment of the hallux rigidus. Foot Ankle Clin 2005;10:75–96.
29. Van Saase JL, Van Romunde LK, Cats A, et al. Epidemiology of osteoarthritis: Zoetermeer survey. Comparison of radiological osteoarthritis in a Dutch population with that in 10 other populations. Ann Rheum Dis 1989;48:271–80.
30. Smith RW, Katchis SD, Ayson LC. Outcomes in hallux rigidus patients treated nonoperatively: a long-term follow-up study. Foot Ankle Int 2000;21:906–13.
31. Harris TG, Smith RW. Moberg osteotomy. In: Wiesel SW, editor. Operative techniques in orthopaedic surgery. Philadelphia: Lippincott Williams & Wilkins; 2011. p. 3585–91.
32. Hattrup SJ, Johnson KA. Subjective results of hallux rigidus following treatment with cheilectomy. Clin Orthop Relat Res 1988;(226):182–91.
33. Coughlin MJ, Shurnas PS. Hallux rigidus: grading and long-term results of operative treatment. J Bone Joint Surg Am 2003;85:2072–88.
34. Citron N, Neil M. Dorsal wedge osteotomy of the proximal phalanx for hallux rigidus. Long-term results. J Bone Joint Surg Br 1987;69:835–7.
35. Kilmartin TE. Phalangeal osteotomy versus first metatarsal decompression osteotomy for the surgical treatment of hallux rigidus: a prospective study of age-matched and condition-matched patients. J Foot Ankle Surg 2005;44:2–12.

36. Rees R, Hartley RH, Henry AP. Extension osteotomy: a good operation for hallux rigidus. Presented at the British Orthopaedic Foot Surgery Society Meeting. Derby, United Kingdom, November 13–15, 1998.

37. Rochwerger A, Farhat I, Azam F, et al. Joint preserving technique in hallux rigidus: a seven-year follow-up. Presented at the 8th Congress of the European Federation of National Associations of Orthopaedics and Traumatology (EFFORT). Florence, Italy. May 11–15, 2007.

38. Wingenfeld C, Abbara-Czardybon M, Arbab D, et al. Cheilectomy and Kessel-Bonney procedure for treatment of initial hallux rigidus. Oper Orthop Traumatol 2008;20:484–91 [in German].

39. Coughlin MJ, Shurnas PS. Hallux rigidus: surgical techniques (cheilectomy and arthrodesis). J Bone Joint Surg Am 2004;86(1 Suppl 2):119–30.

Resurfacing of the Metatarsal Head to Treat Advanced Hallux Rigidus

Alex J. Kline, MD, Carl T. Hasselman, MD*

KEYWORDS

- Hallux rigidus • Hallux limitus • Arthroplasty • Great toe • HemiCAP • Resurfacing

KEY POINTS

- The HemiCAP prosthesis (Arthrosurface Inc, Franklin, MA, USA) is a novel approach to the treatment of arthritis of the first metatarsophalangeal (MTP) joint because it resurfaces the metatarsal head.
- Impaction of the proximal phalanx on the metatarsal head could be a major cause for pain generation in hallux rigidus.
- Hemiarthroplasty techniques that resurface the proximal phalanx still leave a damaged metatarsal head surface.
- The impaction of the implant onto the remaining damaged metatarsal head could be a major cause for persistent pain with those implants.
- Adequate soft tissue release and achieving appropriate alignment intraoperatively are imperative.

INTRODUCTION

Hallux rigidus is a progressive arthritic disorder of the first MTP joint causing pain, loss of motion, and enlargement of the joint.[1,2] When nonoperative management has failed, surgical procedures such as cheilectomy[3,4] and several osteotomies[5,6] may be suitable for stage 1 and 2 hallux rigidus. However, these procedures are not effective for the treatment of more advanced stages.[7] Resection arthroplasty,[8,9] interpositional arthroplasty,[10–12] hemiarthroplasty,[13,14] total joint arthroplasty,[15,16] and arthrodesis[17–19] have all been used for more advanced stages of the disease. Each of these procedures has its own benefits and deficits.

Hemiarthroplasties, which resurface the proximal phalangeal base, have shown promise, but stiffness, continued joint pain, and prosthetic loosening are the limitations to these techniques.[13,14] Arthrodesis has been advocated by many investigators

Dr C.T. Hasselman is a paid consultant for Arthrosurface Inc, Arthrex, and Small Bones Innovations. Dr A.J. Kline is a paid consultant for Arthrex.
University of Pittsburgh Medical Center, Three Rivers Orthopaedic Associates, 200 Delafield Road, Suite 1040, Pittsburgh, PA 15215, USA
* Corresponding author.
E-mail address: hasselmanct@upmc.edu

for treating advanced hallux rigidus,[18–20] and a recent study showed outcomes of arthrodesis after 30 months of follow-up to be superior to those of metallic hemiarthroplasties that resurface the phalangeal base with 79.4 months follow-up.[21] However, limitations in shoe wear, transfer metatarsalgia, permanent limitations in activity, prolonged recovery, and complications from malrotation, malpositioning, malunion, or nonunion have made this procedure less attractive to the younger, active patient.[1,2,22–25]

The HemiCAP was introduced to resurface damaged articular surfaces. The concept is to use intraoperative joint mapping and implantation of a matching, congruent resurfacing prosthesis to allow for joint preservation and restoration of the normal geometry. The procedure has been described in the shoulder, hip, and knee with good clinical outcomes.[26–28] Since 2004, this technology has been used to resurface the metatarsal head in the treatment of advanced hallux rigidus (**Fig. 1**). The technique and initial experiences with this implant have been presented and published in the past.[29–31] This article focuses on the techniques, pearls, postoperative management, and results of metatarsal head resurfacing for advanced hallux rigidus.

INDICATIONS

Metatarsal head resurfacing is performed in those patients who have stage 2 or 3 hallux rigidus who have failed conservative treatment and wish to have an active lifestyle. Resurfacing of the metatarsal head will not benefit patients with inflammatory connective tissue diseases (such as rheumatoid arthritis) or crystalline diseases such as gout or pseudogout. Patients with sesamoid arthritis may not benefit from this procedure unless other techniques are also used to address the sesamoid pain (discussed later in the article). Individuals who have clinically significant peripheral neuropathy and lack protective sensation should not have this procedure done. Patients who have stage 1 hallux rigidus with mostly normal cartilage on the metatarsal head are best treated with a cheilectomy or biological procedure. With these exceptions, all others are candidates for metatarsal head resurfacing.

SURGICAL TECHNIQUE
Preoperative Planning

Preoperative disease severity can be graded according to the classification of Hattrup and Johnson[32] (**Table 1**). Standardized weight-bearing anteroposterior, oblique, and lateral radiographs of the foot should be obtained before surgery. The joint should be evaluated for the degree of arthritis including the loss of joint space, the presence

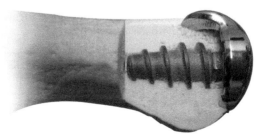

Fig. 1. The HemiCAP dorsiflexion implant for resurfacing the metatarsal head of the first MTP joint. The taper post provides immediate rigid fixation of the implant. (*Courtesy of* Arthrosurface, Franklin, MA.)

Table 1 Hattrup and Johnson radiographic classification		
		N
Grade 1	Mild to moderate osteophyte formation but good joint space preservation	0
Grade 2	Moderate osteophyte formation with joint space narrowing and subchondral sclerosis	16 (53%)
Grade 3	Marked osteophyte formation and loss of visible joint space with or without subchondral cyst formation	14 (47%)

From Hattrup SJ, Johnson KA. Subjective results of hallux rigidus following treatment with cheilectomy. Clin Orthop Relat Res 1988;226:184; with permission.

of osteophytes, subchondral cysts, and sesamoid arthritis. Additional factors to evaluate for radiographically include[33] elevation of the first ray[34] and declination angle of the first metatarsal.[35] Radiographs should also be assessed for an increase in the intermetatarsal angle between the first and second metatarsal. If any of these deformities exist, then they should be addressed with fusions, proximal metatarsal osteotomies, or other techniques to reduce the deformities present. These additional procedures can be done before the resurfacing or at the time of the resurfacing technique. A preoperative computed tomographic scan could evaluate the degree of sesamoid arthritis in the MTP joint and can allow the surgeon to determine if techniques to resurface the sesamoid articulation such as an interpositional arthroplasty as described by Berlet and colleagues[10] or a primary fusion should be performed. In the senior author's (Dr. Hasselman) experience the technique of Berlet and colleagues[10] could be combined with metatarsal head resurfacing to address sesamoid arthritis; however, the other option would be primary fusion of the MTP joint.

Physical examination should ensure an adequate soft tissue envelope over the metatarsal head to allow for adequate healing. Any concerns with the vascular status of the foot should also be addressed before surgery. Sensory testing of the foot with Semmes-Weinstein monofilament testing should ensure normal protective sensation. There are no age limitations for this implant, and the preoperative range of motion has not been found to have any effect on postoperative results. The sesamoid articulation should be assessed by direct palpation while manually dorsiflexing the toe to ensure that this articular surface is not a major source of the patient's symptoms. If the sesamoids seem to be involved in the arthritic process, then other procedures along with the HemiCAP or arthrodesis should be planned; however, sesamoid involvement with the arthritic process is not an absolute contraindication to this technique.

Surgical Procedure

The patient is placed in a supine position on the operating table with the operative extremity in a well-padded position. The procedure can be done with either a regional block and a calf tourniquet or an ankle block with an Esmarch bandage wrapped around the ankle. A dorsal incision is made over the first MTP joint and slightly medial to the extensor hallucis longus tendon. The subcutaneous tissues are spread gently to expose the dorsal joint capsule with care to protect the dorsomedial branch of the superficial peroneal nerve. The extensor hallucis tendon is freed from the capsule and retracted laterally to keep the tendon within its sheath if possible. A longitudinal arthrotomy is made along the medial border of the joint with the incision as medial as possible but avoiding injury to the dorsomedial branch of the superficial peroneal nerve. The capsule and collateral ligaments are released off the metatarsal head with subperiosteal dissection similar to what is done with total knee arthroplasty. The collateral ligaments, sesamoid suspension ligaments, and capsule should be completely released so that the entire joint, including the sesamoids, is easily visualized (**Fig. 2**).

It is very important to visualize the cristae of the sesamoid articulation because this is the landmark for sizing of the implant. In advanced hallux rigidus, the sesamoids and flexor hallucis brevis have fibrotic adhesions to the metatarsal head, which limits dorsiflexion (DF) postoperatively. Care should be taken to avoid damaging the sesamoid articulation with the plantar metatarsal head. The insertions of the plantar plate and flexor hallucis brevis tendon are then released from the proximal portion of the proximal phalanx using subperiosteal dissection similar to a hamstring release in a contracted knee joint when doing knee replacement (**Fig. 3**). This step has a similar effect in the sense that it will release the contracture but allow for the tendons and plantar plate to reattach in a less-contracted position. As the bone remains in place, the tendons scar down or reinsert into the remaining proximal phalanx. There are strips of the flexor hallucis brevis that attach to the flexor hallucis longus, which will hold the tendon in its proper orientation until it can secure itself back to the bone of the proximal phalanx. From experience of performing over 500 implant surgeries, it is the opinion of the senior author that if 90° of dorsiflexion of the first MTP joint has not been achieved with the ankle in neutral dorsiflexion at the completion of the operation, to include implant positioning, then further soft tissue release is needed to ensure adequate postoperative motion.

Once the joint is exposed and adequate soft tissue release is completed, resurfacing of the metatarsal head is completed in a stepwise manner as described by the manufacturer (Arthrosurface). A drill guide is used to place a pin within the shaft of the first metatarsal using a guide on the implant set. Often, wear of the metatarsal head is asymmetrical and so the pin needs to be placed within the center of the metatarsal shaft in both the sagittal and coronal planes. Fluoroscopy may be needed to verify adequate position of the pin. A cannulated double-step drill is inserted over the guide wire, and the metatarsal head is drilled until the proximal shoulder of the drill is flush with the plantar articular surface of the metatarsal head.

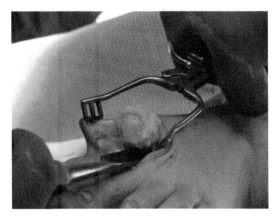

Fig. 2. The entire metatarsal head is degloved for 2 cm proximal to the joint line to ensure adequate release of the collateral ligaments. The plantar plate is released to the midshaft area to ensure no residual contractures.

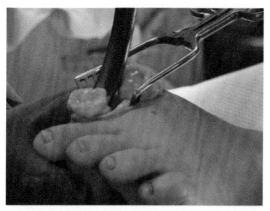

Fig. 3. The insertions of the flexor hallucis brevis and plantar plate are released off the plantar aspect of the proximal phalanx with subperiosteal dissection.

In most instances, the plantar articular surface is the only normal surface, so this surface is used for determination of the depth of the taper post placement. The tap is removed, and the taper post is inserted over the guide wire. The taper post is inserted until the etched line on the driver is flush with the plantar articular surface of the metatarsal head. If one chooses to decompress the joint by slightly shortening the metatarsal, then the taper post is inserted 1 or 2 mm deeper than this. The metatarsal head articular geometry is checked with mapping measuring guides, and the final size of the implant determined. The appropriate implant is chosen, and the metatarsal head resurfaced with 2 reamers to match the shape of the implant. The trail implant is then placed onto the taper post, and the final position of the implant is checked to ensure adequacy of coverage (**Fig. 4**). With the trial implant in place, any bone around the implant is removed from the medial, lateral, and dorsal sides (**Fig. 5**). Once this is completed, the trial implant is removed and the final implant is impacted onto the taper post with gentle blows to lock the morse taper. As stated before, at this point, the range of motion of the MTP joint is tested with the ankle in neutral dorsiflexion. If the first MTP joint does not have the same range of motion as

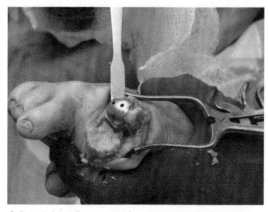

Fig. 4. Placement of the trial implant onto the taper post before to resection of any excess bone.

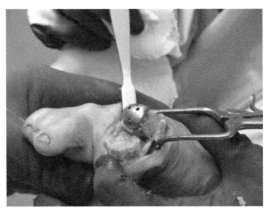

Fig. 5. The trial implant in place and after resection of the excess bone around the trial implant. Note the plantar surface is untouched.

the second MTP joint, then further soft tissue releases are needed until the 2 are equal to ensure adequate postoperative range of motion of the arthroplasty. The key pearls to success with this technique include adequate soft tissue release, addressing sesamoid arthritis, and treating arthrosis of the phalangeal side.

The most common reason for failure is persistent stiffness and pain because of failure of adequate soft tissue release.[36] The metatarsal head must undergo release of all the collateral ligaments so that the entire distal 3 cm of the metatarsal head is completely released of all soft tissue attachments. There is still an intraosseous blood supply so the risk of avascular necrosis (AVN) is minimal. The authors have not seen any in their experience. The proximal phalanx should also be released of its soft tissue attachments. This is a disease of soft tissue contractures on the plantar surface so failure to release these tissues will result in recurrence of pain and stiffness. Cock-up toe or other deformities have not been seen with this aggressive soft tissue release.

Persistent sesamoid arthritis is another concern when resurfacing the metatarsal head.[36] Once the implant is in place, sesamoid arthritis can be addressed by placing a soft tissue graft between the sesamoids and plantar metatarsal head using a "boxing glove" technique as described by Berlet and colleagues[10] The graft is placed over the implant on the metatarsal head and covers the entire remaining articular surface of the plantar metatarsal and sutured in place.

For significant arthritis of the phalangeal base, there are now 2 options. In the first option, the cheilectomy is performed at the phalangeal base and the dorsal capsule of the first MTP joint is transferred to the base of the proximal phalanx (**Fig. 6**).[30] In the other option, the phalangeal side is resurfaced with an implant. The ToeMotion (Arthrosurface) is a metal-backed polyethylene implant designed to resurface the proximal phalangeal side if the disease has progressed significantly to this area (**Fig. 7**). Results of this implant are pending, and long-term results are not yet available. The various technical aspects of this surgery and their benefits for implant success are summarized in **Table 2**.

Postoperative Care

Patients are instructed to begin immediate full weight bearing on the foot, they are shown how to do passive range of motion of the great toe, which begins on postoperative day 1. The motion exercises are to be done a minimum of 5 times a day for

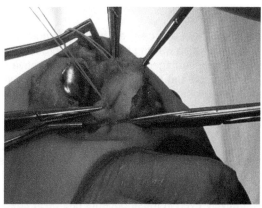

Fig. 6. A portion of the dorsal capsule is being attached to the proximal phalanx using 2 absorbable suture anchors.

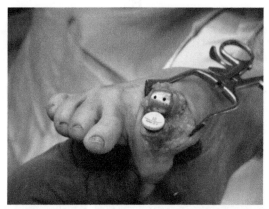

Fig. 7. The phalangeal side has been resurfaced with a metal-backed polyethylene surface, which is secured to the phalangeal with a taper post as in the metatarsal head.

Table 2	
Summary of technical and clinical considerations	
Considerations	**Clinical Goal**
Aggressive soft tissue release	Exposure, range of motion
Joint decompression by altering the joint line: advancing the fixation component 1–3 mm	Range of motion, pain relief
Subperiosteal release of fibrotic flexor brevis tendon at its insertion	Range of motion
Release of sesamoid adhesions to include proximal plantar plate release at its insertion	Range of motion
Metatarsal cheilectomy	Range of motion
Proximal phalanx resurfacing with capsular interpositional graft in bipolar degeneration of more than 50% of the phalangeal surface	Pain relief
Nonmetal fixation for phalangeal concomitant procedures (correctional osteotomies, interpositional graft fixation) to avoid metalosis	Avoid complications
Aggressive and early postoperative mobilization to maximize intraoperative gain in range of motion	Range of motion

10 to 15 minutes each time. These exercises are walking without a postoperative shoe on when at home and focusing on walking heel to toe in order to force motion of the hallux. Ice and elevation are encouraged for the first postoperative week. At 2 weeks, patients begin physical therapy and are encouraged to wear regular shoes as tolerated. Running, impact exercises, and high-heeled shoes are allowed at 6 weeks postoperatively (**Fig. 8**).

Complications

As with surgery on any joint, the potential complications include persistent pain, stiffness, infection, and neurologic injury. With this particular technique, the most common complication has been loss of the intraoperative dorsiflexion; however, the range of motion seen postoperatively even in these patients has been adequate and without

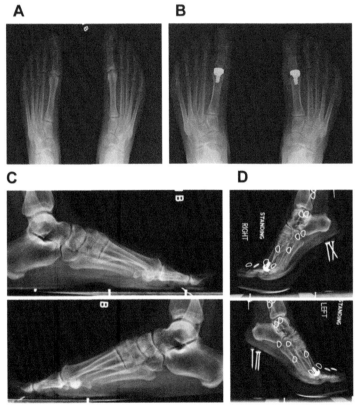

Fig. 8. (*A*) Preoperative weight-bearing anteroposterior (AP) radiographs of a patient with moderate bilateral hallux rigidus who refused fusion as an option to her disease. (*B*) Postoperative weight-bearing AP radiographs of the same woman 2 months after hemiarthroplasties. (*C*) Preoperative weight-bearing lateral radiographs in the patient in **Fig. 5**. Note that the stiffness of her first MTP has caused hyperextension at the distal interphalangeal joint of each great toe to allow for more motion. (*D*) Postoperative weight-bearing lateral radiographs in the patient in **Fig. 5**. Note that the motion of the first MTP has allowed significant improvements in shoe wear. The sesamoids move with the toe, even though she had a flexor hallucis brevis tendon release and plantar plate stripping. The hyperextension of the interphalangeal has resolved because of increased motion at the MTP joint.

Table 3 SF-36 health survey with RAND calculation scores			
Component (N = 26)	Preoperative	Postoperative	P Value
Physical Functioning (1)	66.4	95.2	<.001
Role: Physical (1)	67.3	99.0	<.001
Bodily Pain (1)	60.7	90.2	<.001
Social Functioning (2)	79.98	97.25	<.001
Mental Health (2)	77.2	79.98	.21
Role: Emotional (2)	79.9	97.4	<.001
Vitality (2)	65.96	69.6	.075
General Health (1)	72.7	77.9	.001
Physical Health Component (1)	66.7	90.6	<.001
Mental Health Component (2)	75.8	85.8	<.001

activity limitations. On rare occasions, patients have gone for a manipulation under anesthesia, much as is done with a stiff total knee. Other complications have been delayed wound healing and superficial infections, which have responded to local wound care and oral antibiotics. Sometimes patients have plantar pain for several months after this procedure either from mild sesamoid arthritis or from the plantar soft tissues needing to heal. This pain usually resolves within a 4- to 6-month period. Nonsteroidal antiinflammatory drugs can help to alleviate the pain until resolution.

OUTCOMES

Patients have been assessed preoperatively and at intervals over the postoperative period using the 36-Item Short Form 36 Health Survey (SF-36)[37–40] and the American Orthopedic Foot and Ankle Society (AOFAS) clinical rating system for the hallux.[41] The results of this technique have been published on numerous occasions.[29–31] The average time for return to work was 7 days. Range of motion assessment, AOFAS scores, and visual analog scores all significantly improved from preoperative values. The SF-36 data showed significant improvements in all areas except mental health (**Table 3**). Although the reported studies show significant improvement in most areas, the length of these studies would be considered medium follow-up (range of 5–7 years), and long-term studies with this implant of 10 years or more are pending.

SUMMARY

The HemiCAP prosthesis is a novel approach to the treatment of arthritis of the first MTP joint because it resurfaces the metatarsal head. Studies have shown a better range of motion, greater pain reduction, and higher patient satisfaction with this technique when compared with the other implant hemiarthroplasties.[13,14] One possible explanation is that the metatarsal head is usually the more involved side of the MTP joint degeneration in hallux rigidus. Resurfacing the metatarsal side would therefore address the more-advanced cartilage destruction and provide better pain relief. Furthermore, impaction of the proximal phalanx on the metatarsal head could be a major causal factor for pain generation in hallux rigidus. Hemiarthroplasty techniques that resurface the proximal phalanx still leave a damaged metatarsal head surface. The impaction of the implant onto the remaining damaged metatarsal head could be a major cause for persistent pain with those implants. Technically the implant can be advanced further into the metatarsal head by several millimeters allowing for decompression of the joint and reduction of impact forces. This technique of decompressing the joint has been previously described by others as a means of relieving joint stresses.[2,5,29]

In the authors' series of over 500 cases there has been no evidence of implant loosening or osteolysis around the HemiCAP implant to date. They also found no evidence of radiolucent implant loosening, subsidence, or disengagement. In contrast, loosening of the implant is a significant problem even with short-term follow-up of hemiarthroplasty implants that resurface the proximal phalanx.[13,14] Other metatarsal implants that have appeared since the HemiCAP have also shown subsidence and loosening. It is possible that the shear stresses seen in the proximal phalanx or metatarsal head with repetitive dorsiflexion and weight bearing cause the implant to loosen or prevent proper bony ingrowth early on. Furthermore, shear stresses typically experienced by onlay implants are reduced for the HemiCAP implant, which is placed as an inlay onto a supporting bone bed and connected to a tapered screw fixation component. Early rigid fixation of the implant with a taper post may be the key to prevent subsidence in implants for the first MTP. Even patients with AVN of the metatarsal head from other procedures have been treated with this implant since the post usually bypasses the area of AVN and provides secure fixation of the implant into normal bone. This experience alone suggests that the taper post provides rigid fixation deep into the metatarsal head and provides stability to the resurfacing component of the implant.

The authors found that the phalangeal side does appear to undergo dysplastic changes similar to what has been reported for the acetabulum with hemiarthroplasty of the hip joint. Although the phalangeal side showed changes in most people, few were symptomatic. Since the introduction of the HemiCAP 10 years ago, the authors have seen this phenomenon in approximately 5% of the patients. Those who are symptomatic have gone on to either a successful fusion or phalangeal-sided revision with the ToeMotion prosthesis.

It remains important to stress the risks and pitfalls associated with MTP arthrodesis when comparing treatment options for advanced hallux rigidus. Several complications have been reported with this procedure, including nonunion, transfer metatarsalgia,[1,42,43] progressive interphalangeal (IF) irritation and degeneration,[1,43,44] difficulty with kneeling and other activities,[44] as well as marked changes in gait pattern and foot function.[44–47] Malalignment is also a major pitfall after arthrodesis.[42] It is critical to achieve neutral rotation, adequate dorsiflexion, and adequate valgus while keeping in mind that too little valgus places the interphalangeal joint at risk of degenerative arthritis, whereas excessive valgus may cause difficulty in shoe wear. Excessive dorsiflexion may cause pressure on the dorsal aspect of the toe, whereas inadequate dorsiflexion may create pressure on the tip of the toe.[42] In addition, inadequate joint preparation could lead to a nonunion or fibrous union. In the presence of sclerotic bone, meticulous joint preparation requires reaming and debridement to cancellous bone surfaces to enable a successful arthrodesis.[42] Given these risks and pitfalls, it is ill-fated to endorse fusion as a universally accepted treatment option for patients with stage 2 or 3 hallux rigidus, but it should rather be considered a treatment of final resort and a clinical exit strategy.

Reported measurements of motion during normal gait vary with values for dorsiflexion ranging from 50° to 90°.[48–50] Nawoczenski and colleagues[51] found that measurements of range of motion exceeded the motion that is required during normal walking. The investigators concluded that only 42° ± 2.3° of dorsiflexion was necessary for normal walking gait. In the authors' experience, patients having hemiarthroplasty with the HemiCAP achieved an AROM (active range of motion) of 47.9° thereby also exceeding the requirement for normal gait patterns. When compared with previous reports of hemiarthroplasty and joint fusion, current results of metatarsal head resurfacing demonstrate equivalent or better results for range of motion, pain reduction, and patient satisfaction. The authors have expressed their opinions, techniques, and results in a recent article as well.[36]

REFERENCES

1. Brage ME, Ball ST. Surgical options for salvage of end-stage hallux rigidus. Foot Ankle Clin North Am 2002;7:49–73.
2. Giannini S, Ceccarelli F, Faldini C, et al. What's new in surgical options for hallux rigidus? J Bone Joint Surg Am 2004;86A(Suppl 2):72–83.
3. Mann RA, Clanton TO. Hallux rigidus: treatment by cheilectomy. J Bone Joint Surg Am 1988;70A:400–6.
4. Mulier T, Steenwerckx A, Thienpont E, et al. Results after cheilectomy in athletes with hallux rigidus. Foot Ankle Int 1999;20:232–7.
5. Moberg E. A simple operation for hallux rigidus. Clin Orthop Relat Res 1979;142:55–6.
6. Thomas PJ, Smith RW. Proximal phalanx osteotomy for the surgical treatment of hallux rigidus. Foot Ankle Int 1999;20:3–12.
7. Coughlin MJ, Shurnas PS. Hallux rigidus. Grading and long-term results of operative treatment. J Bone Joint Surg Am 2003;85A:2072–88.
8. Cleveland M, Winant EM. An end-result study of the Keller operation. J Bone Joint Surg Am 1950;32A:163–75.
9. Wrighton JD. A ten-year review of Keller's operation. Review of Keller's operation at the Princess Elizabeth Orthopedic Hospital, exeter. Clin Orthop Relat Res 1972;89:207–14.
10. Berlet GC, Hyer CF, Lee TH, et al. A soft-tissue interpositional arthroplasty technique of the first metatarsophalangeal joint for the treatment of advanced hallux rigidus using a human acellular dermal regenerative tissue matrix. Tech Foot Ankle Surg 2006;5:257–65.
11. Kennedy JG, Chow FY, Dines J, et al. Outcomes after interpositional arthroplasty for treatment of hallux rigidus. Clin Orthop Relat Res 2006;445:210–5.
12. Miller SD. Interposition resection arthroplasty for hallux rigidus. Tech Foot Ankle Surg 2004;3:158–64.
13. Giza E, Sullivan MR. First metatarsophalangeal hemiarthroplasty for grade III and IV hallux rigidus. Tech Foot Ankle Surg 2005;4:10–7.
14. Townley CO, Taranow WS. A metallic hemiarthroplasty resurfacing prosthesis for the hallux metatarsophalangeal joint. Foot Ankle Int 1994;15:575–80.
15. Fuhrmann RA. MTP prosthesis (Reflexion) for hallux rigidus. Tech Foot Ankle Surg 2005;4:2–9.
16. Johnson KA, Buck PG. Total replacement arthroplasty of the first metatarsophalangeal joint. Foot Ankle 1981;1:307–14.
17. Gibson JN, Thomson CE. Arthrodesis or total replacement arthroplasty for hallux rigidus: a randomized controlled trial. Foot Ankle Int 2005;26:680–90.
18. Mann RA, Oates JC. Arthrodesis of the first metatarsophalangeal joint. Foot Ankle 1980;1:159–66.
19. Smith RW, Joanis TL, Maxwell PD. Great toe metatarsophalangeal joint arthrodesis: a user friendly technique. Foot Ankle 1992;13:367–77.
20. Fitzgerald JA, Wilkinson JM. Arthrodesis of the metatarsophalangeal joint of the great toe. Clin Orthop Relat Res 1981;157:70–7.

21. Raikin SM, Ahmad J, Pour AE, et al. Comparison of Arthrodesis and Metallic Hemiarthroplasty of the Hallux Metatarsophalangeal Joint. J Bone J Surg Am 2007;89:1979–85.

22. Coughlin MJ. Arthrodesis of the first metatarsophalangeal joint. Orthop Rev 1990; 19:177–86.

23. Fitzgerald JA. A review of long-term results of arthrodesis of the first metatarsophalangeal joint. J Bone Joint Surg Am 1969;51A:488–93.

24. Hamilton WG, O'Malley MJ, Thompson FM, et al. Capsular interpositional arthroplasty for severe hallux rigidus. Foot Ankle Int 1997;18:68–70.

25. Henry AP, Waugh W, Wood H. The use of footprints in assessing the results of operations for hallux valgus: a comparison of Keller's operation and arthrodesis. J Bone Joint Surg Am 1975;57:478–81.

26. Becher C, Kalbe C, Thermann H, et al. Minimum 5 year results of focal articular prosthetic resurfacing for the treatment of full –thickness articular cartilage defects in the knee. Arch Orthop Trauma Surg 2011;131:1135–43.

27. Jager M, Begg MJ, Krauspe R. Partial hemi-resurfacing of the hip joint – a new approach to treat local osteochondral defects? Biomed Tech 2006;51:371–6.

28. Uribe JW, Botto-van Bemden A. Partial humeral head resurfacing for osteonecrosis. J Should Elbow Surg 2009;18:711–6.

29. Carpenter B, Smith J, Motley T, et al. Surgical treatment of hallux rigidus using a metatarsal head resurfacing implant: mid-term follow-up. J Foot Ankle Surg 2010; 49:321–5.

30. Hasselman CT, Shields N. Resurfacing of the first metatarsal head in the treatment of hallux rigidus. Tech Foot Ankle Surg 2008;7:31–40.

31. Kline AJ, Hasselman CT. Metatarsal head resurfacing for advanced hallux rigidus. Foot Ankle Int 2013;34(5):716–25.

32. Hattrup SJ, Johnson KA. Subjective results of hallux rigidus following treatment with cheilectomy. Clin Orthop Relat Res 1988;226:182–91.

33. Coughlin MJ, Shurnas PS. Soft-tissue arthroplasty for hallux rigidus. Foot Ankle Int 2003;24:661–71.

34. Horton GA, Park YW, Myerson MS. Role of metatarsus primus elevatus in the pathogenesis of hallux rigidus. Foot Ankle Int 1999;20:777–80.

35. Bryant A, Tinley P, Singer K. A comparison of radiographic measurements in normal, hallux valgus, and hallux limitus feet. J Foot Ankle Surg 2000;39:39–43.

36. Hasselman CT. Metatarsal head resurfacing preserves motion in patients with end stage hallux rigidus. Orthopedics Today 2014;34(7):6–7.

37. Ware JE, Sherbourne CD. The MOS 36-Item Short-Form Health Survey (SF-36): I. Conceptual framework and item selection. Med Care 1992;30:473–83.

38. Gatchel RJ, Mayer T, Dersh J, et al. The association of the SF-36 health status survey with 1-year socioeconomic outcomes in a chronically disabled spinal disorder population. Spine 1999;24:2162–70.

39. Taylor SJ, Taylor AE, Foy MA, et al. Responsiveness of common outcome measures for patients with low back pain. Spine 1999;24:1805–12.

40. Hays RD, Sherbourne CD, Mazel RM. The RAND 36-item health survey 1.0. Health Econ 1993;2:217–27.

41. SooHoo NF, Shuler M, Fleming LL. Evaluation of the validity of the AOFAS clinical rating systems by correlation to the SF-36. Foot Ankle Int 2003;24:50–5.

42. Coughlin MJ, Shurnas PS. Hallux rigidus. J Bone Joint Surg 2004;86-A(Suppl 1(Pt 2)):119–30.

43. Kelikian AS. Technical considerations in hallux metatarsophalangeal arthrodesis. Foot Ankle Clin 2005;10:167–90.

44. Taranow WS, Moutsatson MJ, Cooper JM. Contemporary approaches to stage II and III hallux rigidus: the role of metallic hemiarthroplasty of the proximal phalanx. Foot Ankle Clin 2005;10:713–28.
45. DeFrino PF, Brodsky JW, Pollo FE, et al. First metatarsophalangeal arthrodesis: a clinical, pedobarographic and gait analysis study. Foot Ankle Int 2002;23: 496–502.
46. Fuhrmann RA, Wagne A, Anders JO. First metatarsophalangeal joint replacement: the method of choice for end-stage hallux rigidus? Foot Ankle Clin 2003; 8:711–21.
47. Giza E, Sullivan M, Ocel D, et al. First metatarsophalangeal hemiarthroplasty for hallux rigidus. Int Orthop 2010;34:1193–8.
48. Buell T, Green DR, Risser J. Measurements of first metatarsophalangeal joint range of motion. J Am Podiat Med Assoc 1999;78:439–48.
49. Hopson MM, McPhail TO, Cornwall MW. Motion of the first metatarsophalangeal joint. Reliability and validity of four measurement techniques. J Am Podiat Med Assoc 1995;85:198–205.
50. Sheriff MJ, Bejjami FJ, Kummer FJ. Kinematics of the first metatarsophalangeal joint. J Bone Joint Surg Am 1986;68:392–8.
51. Nawoczenski DA, Baumhauer JF, Umberger BR. Relationship between clinical measurements and notion of the first metatarsophalangeal joint during gait. J Bone Joint Surg Am 1999;81:370–6.

Metatarsophalangeal Joint Fusion: Why and How?

Stefan Rammelt, MD, PhD[a],*, Ines Panzner, MD[a], Thomas Mittlmeier, MD, PhD[b]

KEYWORDS

- Hallux rigidus • Arthritis • Metatarsophalangeal joint • Arthrodesis • Nonunion
- Deformity

KEY POINTS

- Arthrodesis of the first metatarsophalangeal (MTP) joint is indicated in patients with end-stage arthritis of the first MTP joint, and deformity and instability of the great toe; it is a salvage procedure after failed osteotomy, resection, interposition, or joint replacement arthroplasty.
- First MTP joint fusion aims at elimination of pain resulting from end-stage arthritis and obtaining a stable, plantigrade first toe.
- Fusion is mostly obtained with screws, staples, and low-profile plates.
- Complications include infection, osteonecrosis, implant protrusion or failure, nonunion, and malunion (the latter 2 each with rates of ~6%); the medium-term results of first MTP joint fusion indicate mostly good functional results with success rates of approximately 90%.

INTRODUCTION

Arthritis of the first metatarsophalangeal (MTP) joint, also called hallux rigidus or hallux limitus, is a frequent painful forefoot condition that interferes with normal ambulation. It may be caused by joint degeneration, single or repetitive trauma, deformity, neuromuscular conditions, osteochondrosis dissecans, and chronic inflammatory conditions such as gout or rheumatoid arthritis.

The clinical course is characterized by pain, swelling, and restricted dorsiflexion of the great toe. Over time, excessive osteophyte formation (dorsal bunion) will lead to conflict in normal shoewear and further decrease in the range of motion. Depending on the cause, deformities such as hallux valgus, hallux varus, plantarflexion

The authors state that there is no conflict of interest.
[a] Foot & Ankle section, University Center of Orthopaedics and Traumatology, University Hospital Carl Gustav Carus Dresden, Fetscherstrasse 74, Dresden 01307, Germany; [b] Department of Trauma and Reconstructive Surgery, Center of Surgery, University Hospital Rostock, Schillingallee 35, Rostock 18057, Germany
* Corresponding author.
E-mail address: stefan.rammelt@uniklinikum-dresden.de

contracture (hallux flexus), or elevation of the first metatarsal head will be present. Hallux rigidus is commonly graded according to Coughlin and Shurnas.[1] Fusion of the first MTP joint may be considered in grade 3 to 4 end-stage arthritis and after failure of joint-sparing procedures. These late stages are characterized with marked or complete loss of dorsiflexion of the great toe, formation of osteophytes, and substantial loss of cartilage over the first metatarsal head, accompanied by nearly constant pain.

First MTP joint fusion aims at elimination of pain resulting from end-stage arthritis and obtaining a stable, plantigrade first toe.

INDICATIONS AND CONTRAINDICATIONS

Arthrodesis of the first MTP joint is indicated for symptomatic end-stage arthritis. Usually arthrodesis is indicated after a course of nonoperative treatments, which may include nonsteroidal anti-inflammatory drugs, orthoses/insoles, intra-articular injections, shoe modification, foam sleeves, taping, mobilization of great toe and sesamoid bones, strengthening the toe flexor muscles, and stretching the great toe, has been completed without alleviating the symptoms for more than 6 months.[2] It should also be considered in deformities of the great toe in patients with rheumatoid arthritis, neuromuscular diseases, and rigid plantarflexion deformities (eg, after compartment syndrome).[3]

Alternative treatment strategies for end-stage arthritis include resection, interposition, or joint replacement arthroplasty of the first MTP joint. Fusion is an excellent treatment choice for patients with severe deformity or instability. First MTP joint fusion is further indicated after failed joint-preserving osteotomies and after failed resection, interposition, or joint replacement arthroplasty.[4]

First MTP joint fusion should not be the first treatment option in early-stage hallux rigidus if cheilectomy or joint-preserving osteotomies are feasible. In cases of compromised soft tissues, such as chronic ulceration and infection, and complicated diabetes mellitus, amputation of the great toe should be considered. Caution is warranted with rigid scar formation after previous surgery, especially with direct adhesion of the skin to the bone (**Table 1**).

SURGICAL TECHNIQUE AND PROCEDURE
Preoperative Planning

- History: pain, trauma, metabolic diseases, shoe conflict, previous surgery
- Inspection of patient's shoewear
- Clinical examination (**Fig. 1**): visible deformities, swelling, palpable dorsal osteophyte (bunion), callus formation, ulcerations, reddening, pre-existing scars, active/passive range of motion and/or instability in the first MTP joint, first-ray elevation, hypermobility of first tarsometatarsal and/or interphalangeal joints, flexible or fixed lesser toe deformities, neuromuscular and vascular deficits, numbness/dysesthesia over the medial sensory nerve
- Radiographic evaluation (**Fig. 2**): standing dorsoplantar (anteroposterior [AP]), lateral, and sesamoid radiographs, being alert to overall foot configuration, deformities, joint-space narrowing, osteophytes, sesamoid hypertrophy, elevated first ray
- Further examinations as needed for special indications: MRI or single-photon emission computed tomography for suspected chronic infection or avascular necrosis. A computed tomography scan may be useful in selected cases to determine the amount of bone loss or if osteoarthritis at the sesamoids is suspected

Table 1
Indications and contraindications for first MTP joint fusion

Indications	Contraindications
Grade 4 hallux rigidus	Grade 1–2 hallux rigidus
Grade 3 hallux rigidus with ≥50% loss of articular cartilage, marked deformity	Grade 3 hallux rigidus with <50% loss of articular cartilage
Failed joint-preserving osteotomy	Critical soft-tissue conditions (eg, ulceration, rigid scar formation)
Failed arthroplasty	Recalcitrant, chronic infection (eg, diabetic foot syndrome)
Failed arthrodesis (nonunion)	—
Neuromuscular disorders with loss of active MTP motion	—
Rigid deformity (eg, contracture after compartment syndrome)	—

Preparation and Patient Positioning

- Preoperative cleaning of toes, nails, and interdigital spaces
- Single dose of a broad-spectrum antibiotic (eg, second-generation cephalosporin)
- The patient is placed in a supine position
- The affected foot is prepped 3 times and draped
- If an osseous defect is present, the ipsilateral proximal or distal tibial metaphysis, or iliac crest is draped for autograft retrieval
- A tourniquet is placed at the ipsilateral thigh

Surgical Approach

- Dorsal, longitudinal incision centered over the first MTP joint
- Medial incision in cases of severe scarring over the dorsal aspect; note that a medial approach does not allow for dorsal plating
- Mobilization of the extensor hallucis longus and extensor hallucis brevis tendons

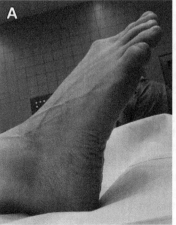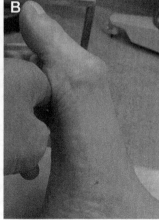

Fig. 1. (*A*, *B*) Clinical appearance of severe hallux rigidus with dorsal bunion and marked limitation of dorsiflexion of the great toe.

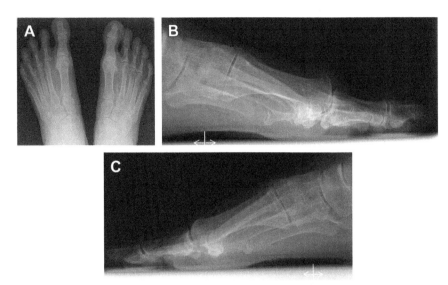

Fig. 2. (*A*) Weight-bearing dorsoplantar (anteroposterior) view of both feet showing marked radiologic joint-space narrowing on the right side. (*B*) Dorsal osteophyte formation and marked elevation of the first metatarsal, compared with the unaffected left side (*C*). Same patient as in **Fig. 1.**

- Careful dissection at the medial and lateral aspect of the first MTP joint with respect the neurovascular bundles

Surgical Procedure

Step 1: preparation of the joint surfaces

- Resection of dorsal, medial, and lateral osteophytes
- Evaluation of the amount of remaining joint cartilage (**Fig. 3**): if more than 50% remaining, joint-sparing procedures may be feasible
- Resection of remaining cartilage and subchondral sclerosis. The preparation of the surfaces depends on the individual bone quality. With soft bone and loose cartilage as occurs in rheumatoid arthritis, the cartilage and subchondral bone can be easily removed with curettes. With hard bone as occurs in severe degenerative osteoarthritis, the use of osteotomes, oscillating saws, or cup-and-cone reamers is preferred
- The use of a cup-in-cone reamer is recommended to achieve a large surface area if the shape of the first metatarsal head and proximal phalanx is still preserved
- Perforating the resected surfaces enhances healing and further enlarges the surface area for fusion (eg, by repetitive drilling with a small-diameter drill (<2.0 mm), Kirschner wire [K-wire], or microfracturing)
- The sesamoids are mobilized; resection is necessary only in case of severe hypertrophy and arthritic changes
- In cases of severe osseous deformity, resection of the joint surfaces aims at achieving good contact for obtaining a solid fusion
- In cases of failed previous fusion, osteotomy, resection, interposition, or implant arthroplasty, all implants, intervening fibrous tissue, and necrotic/sclerotic bone are removed until good-quality bony surfaces are obtained on both the first metatarsal and proximal phalanx

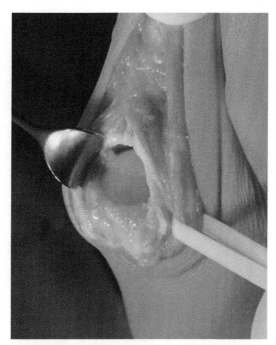

Fig. 3. Intraoperative aspect of a grade 3 hallux rigidus showing complete loss of cartilage of approximately two-thirds of the joint surface. Same patient as in **Figs. 1** and **2**.

- In cases of suspected infection, all avital/infected soft tissue and bone is removed. polymethylmethacrylate cement loaded with antibiotic is interposed as a temporary spacer either as a solid cement block or beads, and fusion with bone grafting is done after eradication of the infection and obtaining sterile specimens from bacteriologic examination

Step 2: defect filling

- Filling of osseous defects aims at achieving a normal length of the first ray and avoiding overload of the second and third metatarsal heads and MTP joints with all the possible consequences
- Remaining defects from resection of sclerotic/necrotic/infected bone are filled with either autologous or homologous bone grafts or bone substitutes. In the authors' practice, autologous bone grafting is preferred (**Fig. 4**)
- Small defects may be filled with cancellous bone from the calcaneus, distal, or proximal tibial metaphysis
- Larger defects are filled with corticocancellous grafting from the anterior iliac crest
- After failed first MTP joint replacement, the defects from removing the prosthesis may be filled with a strut bone graft from the iliac crest (alternatively allograft) that has a double-cone shape to achieve an intrinsic stability for fusion (**Fig. 5**)

Step 3: realignment and internal fixation

- The great toe is positioned in dorsal extension of 10° to 15° and a physiologic valgus position of 5° to 25°.[2,4]

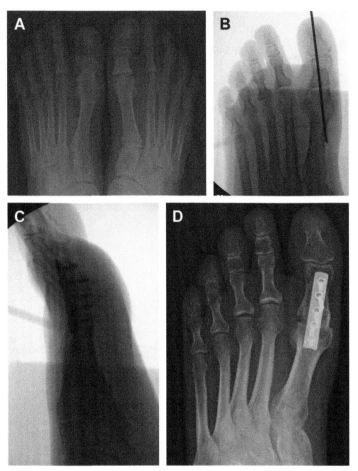

Fig. 4. (*A*) Failed resection arthroplasty with a painful, floppy great toe and shortening of the first ray on the left side. (*B*) Salvage consists of debridement and interposition bone grafting. (*C*) Fixation is achieved with a low-profile plate. (*D*) Weight-bearing dorsoplantar radiograph 6 months after correction, showing solid fusion.

- To achieve an optimal position for the individual patient, the great toe should be aligned parallel to the second toe. The sole of the foot is placed on a flat surface to simulate weight bearing and the pulp of the great toe should slightly touch the surface.[5] In the frontal plane, the nail should be parallel to the ground to avoid malrotation.
- After obtaining the correct length, rotation, and alignment, the first MTP joint is temporarily fixed with 1 or 2 K-wires (**Fig. 6**).
- The correct position is checked by intraoperative dorsoplantar (AP), lateral, and oblique fluoroscopic views.
- Fixation can be achieved with various implants for several indications,[2,4,6] such as the following:
  - Low-profile nonlocking or interlocking plates or combinations of plate and screw(s) for poor bone quality or marked deformity (**Fig. 7**). Biomechanically,

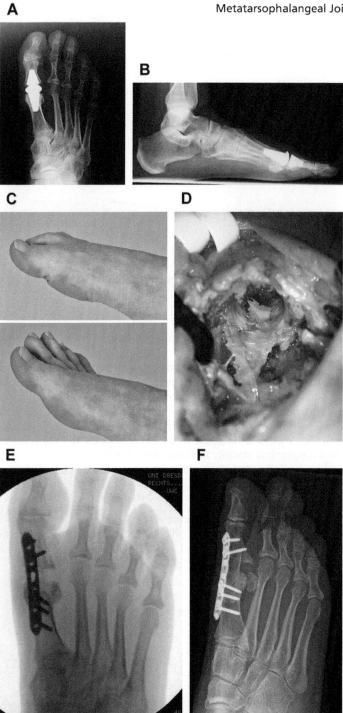

Fig. 5. (*A, B*) Symptomatic loosening of a first MTP joint replacement. The 51-year-old female patient has pain with every step. (*C*) Active motion of the great toe is severely restricted. (*D*) Intraoperative aspect of the first metatarsal after removal of the prosthesis. (*E*) Fusion is achieved without loss of length with an interposition strut bone graft that is cone-shaped toward both the metatarsal and phalangeal side. (*F*) An oblique radiograph 3 months later demonstrates solid fusion. One year after fusion, the patient is walking and free of pain.

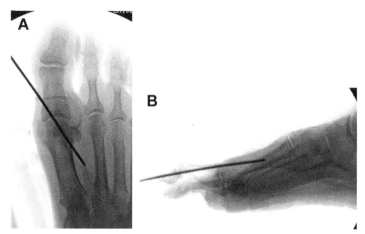

Fig. 6. (*A*, *B*) Fluoroscopic control of alignment after resection of the joint surfaces. Same patient as in **Figs. 1–3**.

the use of a compression lag screw with a dorsal neutralization plate is the most stable construct[5,7,8]

- Interlocking plates with interposition bone grafting for bone defects. Interlocking plates exhibited less plantar gapping and a greater stiffness in load-to-failure testing in a biomechanical investigation[9]
- Two crossed screws, combination of screw and K-wire, or bone clamps for arthritis with normal configuration of the MTP joint and bone quality (**Fig. 8**)
- Other fixation methods include K-wires and wire loops, but these are associated with less mechanical stability than the aforementioned.[5,7]
- Accompanying lesser toe deformities are addressed as indicated.

Postoperative Care

- Gauze and tape dressing postoperatively
- Mobilization in a special shoe with offloading of the forefoot and heel contact for 6 weeks

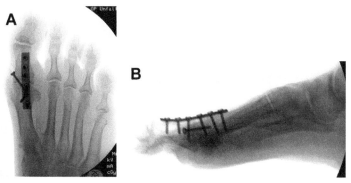

Fig. 7. (*A*, *B*) Fusion is achieved with a low-profile, nonlocking, one-third tubular 2.7-mm plate and one 2.7-mm screw. Same patient as in **Figs. 1–3** and **6**.

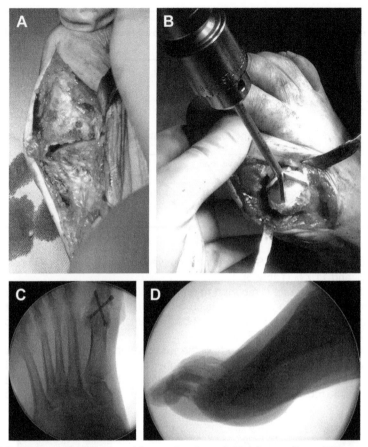

Fig. 8. (*A*) Grade 4 hallux rigidus with complete loss of the joint cartilage. (*B*) Preparing the joint surfaces with cup-and-cone reamers. (*C, D*) First MTP joint fusion is achieved with crossed screws.

- With poor bone stock, partial weight bearing in a cast shoe (Lopresti slipper) or an orthosis with 20 kg is preferred
- After interposition bone grafting, offloading or partial weight bearing for 10 to 12 weeks in a Lopresti slipper is recommended

COMPLICATIONS AND MANAGEMENT

Considering the most frequent complications, a review of 2818 feet from 37 studies found a nonunion rate of 5.4%, a malunion rate of 6.1%, and the need for hardware removal in 8.5% (**Table 2**).[10]

OUTCOMES

The success rate of first MTP joint fusion in an extensive literature review of 1451 cases was reported as 90% more than 2 decades ago.[2] The results from more recent studies indicate mostly good functional medium-term outcomes, with American

Table 2
Summary of the most frequent complications with possible causes and treatment options

Complication	Possible Causes	Treatment
Malalignment	Inadequate intraoperative control of alignment, inadequate technique, failure of fixation	Osteotomy and realignment
Nonunion	Poor bone stock, inadequate resection of the surfaces, immediate postoperative weight bearing	Resection of the fibrous pseudarthrosis, debridement and drilling, fusion with bone grafting (see **Fig. 9**)
Arthritis of adjacent joints	Malalignment, overload	Correction of MTP malalignment, fusion of adjacent joint(s)
Osteonecrosis, osteitis	Poor bone stock and/or soft-tissue conditions	Implant removal, (repeat) debridement, fusion with bone grafting

Orthopedic Foot and Ankle Society scores between 53 and 90 and revision rates between 0% and 11.7% (**Table 3**).

Patient satisfaction rate is reported to range from 73% to 100%.[22,23] In a prospective clinical study using gait analysis, Brodsky and colleagues[24] found objective improvement in propulsive power, weight-bearing function of the whole foot, and stability during gait after first MTP fusion.

Despite the high number of reports of the surgical treatment of hallux rigidus, most publications fail to fulfill the criteria of higher-level evidence-based medicine.[25] Considering the heterogeneity and methodological limitations of the current body of literature on the topic, a valid comparison of the variants of surgical treatment of hallux

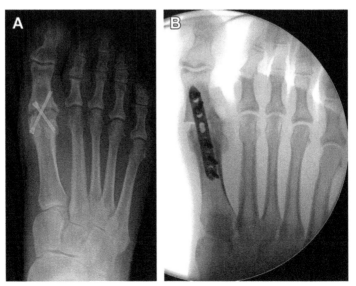

Fig. 9. (*A*) Nonunion after first MTP joint fusion fixed with screws. (*B*) Salvage with repeat debridement and arthrodesis with interposition bone grafting. An interlocking plate is used for fixation.

Table 3
Summary of functional results and revision rates from recent studies on first MTP joint fusion

Authors	Procedures	Follow-Up (y)	AOFAS Postoperatively	Revisions (%)
Lombardi et al,[11] 2001	21	2.4	75.6	4.8
Coughlin & Shurnas,[1] 2003	34	6.7	89	6.6
Ettl et al,[12] 2003	38	4.3	53	0
Gibson & Thomson,[13] 2005	38	2.0	NS	0
Beertema et al,[14] 2006	34	7.0	73	11.7
Raikin et al,[15] 2007	27	6.6	84	0
Bennett and Sabetta,[16] 2009	200	NS	84	1.3
Wassink and van den Oever,[17] 2009	109	5.8	NS	4.6
Kumar et al,[18] 2010	46	1.9	82	2
Kim et al,[19] 2012	51	3.0	90	5.8
Doty et al,[20] 2013	49	<1	77	(2)
Erdil et al,[21] 2013	12	2.7	76	0

Abbreviations: AOFAS, American Orthopedic Foot and Ankle Society score; NS, not stated.

rigidus is impossible, making further adequately powered controlled and randomized studies necessary.[23]

A recent meta-analysis found fair evidence (grade B recommendation) for MTP fusion as a treatment of hallux rigidus, but only poor evidence (grade C recommendation) for cheilectomy, osteotomy, interposition, resection, and implant arthroplasty.[22]

SUMMARY

Fusion of the first MTP joint is a safe and reliable treatment option for end-stage (grade 3–4) hallux rigidus with considerable loss of joint cartilage, severe deformity, and instability of the great toe. It furthermore serves as a viable salvage procedure after failed joint-preserving osteotomy, resection, interposition, or joint replacement arthroplasty. The main treatment goals are elimination of pain and obtaining a stable, plantigrade first toe. Associated deformities are corrected, and greater defects are filled with interposition autograft or allograft. Stable fusion can be achieved with screws, staples, low-profile plates, or a combination of these implants. Complications include infection, osteonecrosis, implant protrusion or failure, nonunion, and malunion. The medium-term results of first MTP joint fusion from the reported studies indicate mostly good functional results, with success and patient satisfaction rates of approximately 90%.

REFERENCES

1. Coughlin MJ, Shurnas PS. Hallux rigidus. Grading and long-term results of operative treatment. J Bone Joint Surg 2003;85-A:2072–88.
2. Coughlin MJ. Arthrodesis of the first metatarsophalangeal joint. Orthop Rev 1990; 19:177–86.
3. Rammelt S, Zwipp H. Reconstructive surgery after compartment syndrome of the lower leg and foot. Eur J Trauma 2008;34:237–48.

4. Hirose CB, Coughlin MJ, Stevens FR. Arthritis of the foot and ankle. In: Coughlin MJ, Saltzman CR, Anderson JB, editors. Mann's surgery of the foot & ankle. 9th edition. Philadelphia: Elsevier Saunders; 2013. p. 867–1007.
5. Fuhrmann RA. Arthrodesis of the metatarsophalangeal joint in hallux rigidus—an overview. Fuss und Sprunggelenk 2011;9:21–9 [in German].
6. Simpson GA, Hembree WC, Miller SD, et al. Surgical strategies: hallux rigidus surgical techniques. Foot Ankle Int 2011;32:1175–86.
7. Buranosky DJ, Taylor DT, Sage RA, et al. First metatarsophalangeal joint arthrodesis: quantitative mechanical testing of six-hole plate versus crossed screw fixation in cadaveric specimens. J Foot Ankle Surg 2001;40:208–13.
8. Politi J, John H, Njus G, et al. First metatarso-phalangeal joint arthrodesis: a biomechanical assessment of stability. Foot Ankle Int 2003;24:332–7.
9. Hunt KJ, Barr CR, Lindsey DP, et al. Locked versus non-locked plate fixation for first metatarsophalangeal joint arthrodesis: a biomechanical investigation. Foot Ankle Int 2012;33:984–90.
10. Roukis TS. Nonunion after arthrodesis of the first metatarsal-phalangeal joint: a systematic review. J Foot Ankle Surg 2011;50(6):710–3.
11. Lombardi CM, Silhanek AD, Connolly FG, et al. First metatarsophalangeal arthrodesis for treatment of hallux rigidus: a retrospective study. J Foot Ankle Surg 2001;40:137–43.
12. Ettl V, Radke S, Gaertner M, et al. Arthrodesis in the treatment of hallux rigidus. Int Orthop 2003;27:382–5.
13. Gibson JN, Thomson CE. Arthrodesis or total replacement arthroplasty for hallux rigidus: a randomized controlled trial. Foot Ankle Int 2005;26:680–90.
14. Beertema W, Draijer WF, van Os JJ, et al. A retrospective analysis of surgical treatment in patients with symptomatic hallux rigidus: long-term follow-up. J Foot Ankle Surg 2006;45:244–51.
15. Raikin SM, Ahmad J, Pour AE, et al. Comparison of arthrodesis and metallic hemiarthroplasty of the hallux metatarsophalangeal joint. J Bone Joint Surg 2007;89-A: 1979–85.
16. Bennett GL, Sabetta J. First metatarsal-phalangeal joint arthrodesis: evaluation of plate and screw fixation. Foot Ankle Int 2009;30:752–9.
17. Wassink S, van den Oever M. Arthrodesis of the first meta-tarsophalangeal joint using a single screw: retrospective analysis of 109 feet. J Foot Ankle Surg 2009; 48:653–61.
18. Kumar S, Pradhan R, Rosenfeld PF. First metatarsophalangeal joint arthrodesis using a dorsal plate and a compression screw. Foot Ankle Int 2010;31:797–801.
19. Kim PJ, Hatch D, DiDomenico LA, et al. A multicenter retrospective review of outcomes for arthrodesis, hemi-metallic joint implant and resectional arthroplasty in the surgical treatment of end-stage hallux rigidus. J Foot Ankle Surg 2012;51: 50–6.
20. Doty J, Coughlin MJ, Hiorose C, et al. Hallux metatarsophalangeal joint arthrodesis with a hybrid locking plate and a plantar neutralization screw: a prospective study. Foot Ankle Int 2013;34:1535–40.
21. Erdil M, Elmadağ NH, Gökhan P, et al. Comparison of arthrodesis, resurfacing hemiarthroplasty and total joint replacement in the treatment of advanced hallux rigidus. J Foot Ankle Surg 2013;52:588–93.
22. Maffulli N, Papalia R, Palumbo A, et al. Quantitative review of operative management of hallux rigidus. Br Med Bull 2011;98:75–98.
23. McNeil DS, Baumhauer JF, Glazebrook MA. Evidence-based analysis of the efficacy for operative treatment of hallux rigidus. Foot Ankle Int 2013;34:15–32.

24. Brodsky JW, Baum BS, Pollo FE. Prospective gait analysis in patients with first metatarsophalangeal joint arthrodesis for hallux rigidus. Foot Ankle Int 2007;28: 162–5.
25. Zammit GV, Menz HB, Munteanu SE, et al. Interventions for treating osteoarthritis of the big toe. Cochrane Database Syst Rev 2010;(9):CD007809.

Metatarsophalangeal Fusion Techniques with First Metatarsal Bone Loss/ Defects

Brian S. Winters, MD[a], Boleslaw Czachor, MD[b],
Steven M. Raikin, MD[b,c],*

KEYWORDS

- First metatarsophalangeal joint fusion • First metatarsal bone loss
- First metatarsal defects • Surgical techniques • Arthrodesis • Revision

KEY POINTS

- A variety of surgical procedures exist for the treatment of first metatarsophalangeal disorder but significant bone loss/defects can result if they go on to failure.
- First metatarsophalangeal joint fusion with tricortical iliac crest bone graft is a viable salvage option for this challenging problem.
- The most important objective with reconstruction is to establish a stable first metatarsophalangeal joint with a balanced metatarsal cascade that reestablishes even forefoot weight-bearing pressures.

INTRODUCTION

First metatarsophalangeal joint (MTPJ) disorder is routinely encountered in the orthopedic clinic and is a major cause of chronic forefoot pain, deformity, and dysfunction.[1]

Several operative procedures have been developed in an attempt to reduce the pain, improve the function, and correct the deformity of these debilitating conditions that affect this versatile joint.[2] These efforts include procedures such as the prosthetic joint replacement (total and hemiarthroplasty), resection arthroplasty (Keller), and

Disclosure: The authors have nothing to disclose.
[a] Rothman Institute for Orthopaedics, 2500 English Creek Blvd, Egg Harbor Township, NJ 08234, USA; [b] Department of Foot and Ankle Surgery, Thomas Jefferson University, The Rothman Institute for Orthopaedics, 1025 Walnut St, Philadelphia, PA 19107, USA; [c] Foot and Ankle Service, Orthopaedic Surgery, Thomas Jefferson University, The Rothman Institute for Orthopaedics, 925 Chestnut Street, Philadelphia, PA 19107, USA
* Corresponding author. Foot and Ankle Service, Orthopaedic Surgery, Thomas Jefferson University, The Rothman Institute for Orthopaedics, 925 Chestnut Street, Philadelphia, PA 19107.
E-mail address: steven.raikin@rothmaninstitute.com

arthrodesis, all of which vary in their success rates. Endoprostheses have been used for nearly 50 years but have yet to gain wide acceptance in the orthopedic community because of the high rates of failure described in the literature. An example of a failed endoprosthesis is shown in **Fig. 1**. Despite improvements in implant design and biomaterials, there remains a high rate of loosening and poor patient satisfaction.[3,4] Resection arthroplasty has been reported to cause excessive shortening of the first ray, which can lead to a weak or floppy toe, cock-up toe deformity, and/or transfer metatarsalgia.[5,6] Arthrodesis continues to be the most successful and reproducible long-term option for reconstruction, with rates of union being described from 56% to 100%.[7–9] However, when a nonunion or malunion does occur, it can be a source of significant pain and dysfunction.

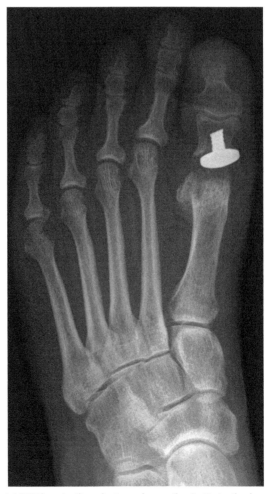

Fig. 1. A failed first MTPJ hemiarthroplasty endoprosthesis. Note the large amount of bone loss around the portion of the implant that is in the proximal phalanx, which implies loosening. There is also severe bone loss on the metatarsal head.

In addition, other surgical procedures can result in a short first metatarsal, resulting in imbalance within the metatarsal cascade, pain, transfer metatarsalgia, and gait dysfunction. A clinical example of a shortened first metatarsal is shown in **Fig. 2**.

MTPJ arthrodesis has been the logical choice for when an arthritic joint is accompanied by severe bone loss or shortening of the first ray.[1,6,9,10] However, significant shortening in the first ray can have severe clinical consequences because approximately 40% to 60% of the body weight passes through the first MTPJ during normal walking and approaches 2 to 3 times this amount during vigorous physical activity, such as jogging or running.[10–12] With marked shortening of the hallux, pain can result in this region and metatarsalgia can subsequently occur as the weight that is usually applied to the MTPJ is transferred laterally to the lesser metatarsal heads. Consequently, the most important objective is to ensure that the final outcome of the corrective procedures is a stable joint with a balanced metatarsal cascade to reestablish even forefoot weight-bearing pressure.

Provided that only mild to moderate bone loss is present, an in situ arthrodesis that leaves the hallux slightly short can be performed,[6] and this is determined by assessing the imbalance of the metatarsal cascade and ensuring that no transfer metatarsalgia results by not addressing the first brachymetatarsal. In general, a discrepancy of less than 5 mm can be fused in situ. This procedure is generally well tolerated because it usually creates minimal cosmetic concerns for patients and affords satisfactory functional improvement in most cases. For moderate shortening (5–10 mm) an in situ arthrodesis can be performed in conjunction with rebalancing of the lesser metatarsal lengths through shortening osteotomies. An example of this is provided in **Fig. 3**, which shows an in situ arthrodesis with a shortening osteotomy of the second and third metatarsals. Resection of the lesser metatarsal heads in this situation should be avoided in order to preserve the anatomy and function as much as possible.[8] An alternative is to perform a joint-sparing shortening osteotomy of the overloaded lesser metatarsals, thereby preserving joint function. This procedure can be performed at various locations within the lesser metatarsals, but is most commonly performed via an oblique sliding osteotomy of the distal metatarsal. However, this method involves operating on otherwise normal joints and can result in additional limitations to the patient. This approach is indicated when there is concomitant deformity (such as a claw

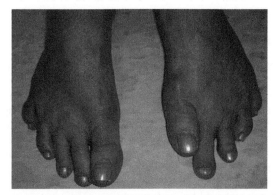

Fig. 2. A clinical example of a shortened first metatarsal. Note the unbalanced metatarsal cascade, which can lead to transfer metatarsalgia caused by abnormal weight bearing on the foot.

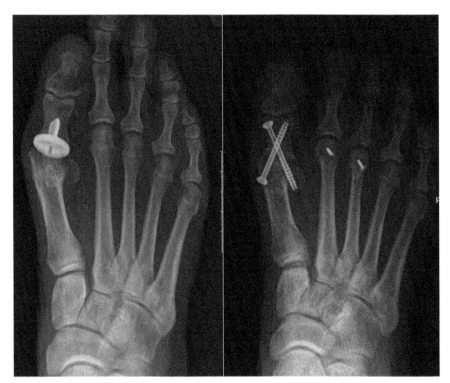

Fig. 3. An in situ arthrodesis performed for first metatarsophalangeal (MTP) bone loss status post a failed hemiarthroplasty implant. Although the fusion accepts a shortened position of the first ray, the second and third metatarsals are concurrently shortened to help rebalance the cascade.

or cross-over deformity) of the lesser MTPJ requiring a corrective osteotomy, which is planned to be done at the same time as the first MTPJ fusion is being performed.

In most cases in which severe bone loss is apparent, the length of the first ray should be reconstructed in order to restore the foot's normal biomechanics and avoid additional pain and dysfunction. This outcome is obtained through performing a bone-block distraction arthrodesis.

INDICATIONS/CONTRAINDICATIONS

Nonoperative treatment is limited for these conditions and primarily includes rigid orthotics and accommodative shoe wear. When any of the various forms of first MTPJ reconstruction go on to failure, revision surgery is indicated if pain, nonunion, and/or instability persist despite these conservative measures. Depending on the amount of bony resection that occurred at the index procedure or is anticipated after debridement of avascular bone in the setting of a failed reconstruction, the surgeon could be presented with a large defect at the time of revision. If there is approximately 1 cm or more of bone loss, and the first metatarsal head is significantly shorter than the remainder of the cascade, a distraction arthrodesis with or without lesser metatarsal shortening osteotomies should be performed in order to restore the proper biomechanics of the foot.[5]

Distraction arthrodesis has a high nonunion rate under ideal circumstances.

Preoperative Planning

The initial step in assessing any patient with pain following a first MTPJ reconstruction includes determining what index procedure has previously been performed. When possible, prior records, including operative reports, documentation of implants used (particularly arthroplasty implants), and preoperative and initial postoperative radiographs, should be requested and obtained from the previous surgeon. These records can be useful in determining the baseline bone quality and length before the initial procedure, and in planning for the revision procedure. A thorough history is obtained as to when the patient began to experience pain, its exact location, and whether any constitutional symptoms are present. A prior history of incision healing difficulties or infection from the initial surgery must be documented.

Physical examination should assess the overall alignment of the foot and ankle because deformity, such as a severe adult-acquired flat foot or valgus ankle, can exacerbate symptoms and further exacerbate pathologic pressure distribution; this may need to be addressed at surgery, either simultaneously or in a staged fashion. If a prior surgery was conducted, scars and skin quality should be carefully evaluated. The distal pulses should be assessed and a vascular consultation obtained if there is any concern for critical peripheral vascular disease. In addition, pain at the lesser metatarsal heads needs to be noted, if present, because transfer metatarsalgia can occur in the setting of a short first ray. Callus formation at the plantar aspect of the metatarsal heads supports this diagnosis. In addition to transfer metatarsalgia, lesser toe metatarsophalangeal (MTP) or proximal interphalangeal joint deformities commonly develop as a result of the abnormal foot biomechanics, and these need to be documented and corrected concomitantly with the first ray.

Weight-bearing anteroposterior (AP), oblique, and lateral radiographs are obtained. These radiographs are inspected to assess for bone loss, osteolysis, prior arthroplasty type and size, or when a prior fusion has been attempted for evidence of a nonunion with or without hardware failure. In addition, the radiographs need to be evaluated for foot alignment, position and alignment of the first MTPJ, for evidence of osteonecrosis of the metatarsal head, as well as the metatarsal cascade. In some situations, advanced imaging modalities, such as MRI and computed tomography, may be needed to further evaluate the underlying disorder and formulate a surgical plan. In cases in which infection is suspected, serologic laboratory studies (erythrocyte Sedimentation rate, C-reactive protein, white cell count) should be performed and a white cell labeled bone scan should be obtained. If these are positive or equivocal, a bone biopsy should be performed before any definitive revision procedure.

After review of all the imaging studies, the surgeon needs to assess the likelihood of encountering significant bone loss at the time of surgery. If a defect is anticipated, a structural autograft or allograft may be needed to properly reconstruct the first ray. The approximate amount of shortening should be estimated preoperatively and adjusted accordingly in the operating room based on the clinical assessment. The graft of choice is typically from the iliac crest because it possesses 3 solid cortices for structural support. Although autograft is preferred to allograft because of its osteoconductive and osteoinductive properties, both have advantages and disadvantages. Harvesting autologous iliac crest bone graft requires a separate surgical procedure that serves as another source of morbidity, such as hematoma, infection, and injury to the lateral femoral cutaneous nerve. Allograft is only osteoconductive and has a theoretic risk, although small, of transmitting disease and malignancy to the recipient. However, Myerson and colleagues[6] reported no cases of disease transmission in their investigation of structural allografts used in foot and ankle surgery.

SURGICAL TECHNIQUE
Prep and Positioning the Patient

Patients should be placed on the operating table in the supine position. If they have significant external rotation of the operative extremity and/or iliac crest autograft is being harvested, a well-padded bump should be placed under the ipsilateral hip so that the foot and iliac crest are easily accessible. If the contralateral hip needs to be accessed for graft harvest, place the bump per your comfort. We recommend using a tourniquet, either a thigh or calf, in order to prevent excessive bleeding into the soft tissues and improve intraoperative visualization. Despite this, meticulous hemostasis needs to be obtained throughout the procedure in order to prevent a postoperative hematoma and reduce the risk of wound complications/infection. The tourniquet can be released at the end of the procedure to accomplish this if necessary. The foot and ankle is then prepped and draped in the standard sterile fashion.

Surgical Approach

Whenever possible, the incision from the prior surgical procedure should be used, even if suboptimally placed, to limited the risk of devascularized skin bridges. The MTPJ is best accessed through a dorsal midline approach, which allows for an expansile incision, if needed, to obtain adequate exposure of the MTPJ. It also avoids the area of the dorsal medial cutaneous nerve, which can be difficult to identify in a revision setting, in which a large amount of scar tissue is usually present. When it is not feasible to use the prior incision, it is best to make the incision as dorsal as possible. The incision should start just distal to the interphalangeal joint and extend proximally enough to gain access to the joint or any implanted hardware that needs to be removed. Therefore the length of the incision varies from patient to patient.

After the skin/subcutaneous tissue is retracted, the extensor hallucis longus (EHL) tendon is encountered and should be retracted laterally. Depending on the amount of shortening at the first ray and/or in the presence of a cock-up hallux deformity, the EHL tendon may need to be lengthened in a Z-type fashion, which can also help gain unrestricted access to the MTPJ. It is subsequently reapproximated at the end of the procedure to reestablish its normal resting tension.

The joint capsule of the MTPJ should then be incised longitudinally in line with the skin incision directly down to bone. The capsule is then released medially and laterally using sharp dissection to open it as a continuous envelope. It is imperative to do this full thickness in order to ensure that sufficient release of the collateral ligaments/scar tissue is obtained and to provide adequate soft tissue coverage during the closure, particularly when a plate is used. The plantar aspect of the joint should be left intact in order to preserve the blood supply to the proximal phalanx and metatarsal. Any osteophytes, remaining soft tissue, and implants are then removed. If the procedure is being performed in the setting of a malunion, then the MTPJ region should be osteotomized with either an osteotome or microsagittal saw accordingly. The joint can now be fully accessed by hyperplantarflexing the joint while retracting the soft tissue with the surgeon's instruments of choice.

Surgical Procedure

Any arthroplasty implant should be removed at this point. In most cases the implant is loose and easily removed. If there are areas of implant ingrowth, great care should be taken to loosen the components without removing additional bone stock. When a Silastic implant is present, large amounts of synovitis are usually present. This synovitis contains numerous macrophages, which results in a persistent inflammatory environment, potentially leading to a nonunion of the fusion, if not adequately debrided and removed. A burr may be beneficial to remove the sclerotic bone and create bleeding bone for fusion, but care must be taken not to overheat the bone and cause thermonecrosis. The proximal phalanx base and metatarsal head are debrided of any necrotic or avascular bone to a healthy, bleeding bed and fashioned in a way that accommodates the interpositional bone graft. This debridement can be done in one of 2 ways: making flat cuts using a microsagittal saw or using MTPJ cup-and-cone reamers. However the graft is prepared, it is important to plan the procedure precisely so that once the graft is put in place, the toe is in an appropriate position with approximately 10° of valgus, neutral rotation, and 10° of dorsiflexion relative to the floor (25° relative to the anatomic declination of the first ray). When using flat cuts, it is best to make these cuts as perpendicular as possible to the long axis of the first ray so that sheer forces can be avoided once the graft is put into position and a stable construct can be obtained. If an acceptable position of the MTPJ is not obtained after the initial cuts, additional cuts are necessary, which places the surgeon at risk of having to deal with further bone loss. While making any bone cuts, the saw blade–bone interface should be irrigated in order to avoid thermal necrosis, which can ultimately result in a nonunion.

Another technique involves using cup-and-cone reamers, which have the advantages of minimizing bone resection and being able to place the toe in multiple different positions while getting complete bony apposition. After the bone ends have been adequately debrided, the diameter of the metatarsal is measured to determine what size reamers should be used. A guidewire (usually supplied with the specific reamers used) is inserted through the center point of the metatarsal head in a retrograde fashion down the center of the shaft. Fluoroscopic guidance is used to ensure that the wire is placed in the center of the metatarsal on both the AP and lateral views to avoid eccentric reaming of the head and additional bone loss. The reamers are extremely aggressive and care should be taken avoid excess bone resection. This process is then repeated on the proximal phalanx side of the MTPJ using the corresponding reamer. Once the MTPJ has been prepared, the toe is pulled into the desired length and position so that the size of the bony defect can be measured. **Fig. 4** shows this intraoperative step. This step determines what size graft needs to be obtained.

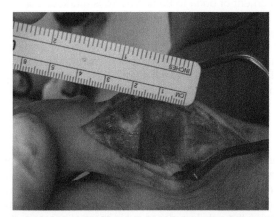

Fig. 4. The intraoperative step in which the clinician places traction on the hallux to determine the amount of bone loss at the first MTPJ. The gap is measured and a graft can be fashioned to fill the defect.

SELECTING THE GRAFT SIZE

It is crucially important to reconstruct the balance of the metatarsal cascade while performing this procedure. In cases of chronic shortening secondary to slow progressive bone loss, associated shortening of the vascular supply to the hallux may occur. If acute lengthening is performed beyond the elasticity of the arterial vessels to compensate for the change in length, ischemia may occur, potentially resulting in loss of the hallux. Once the metatarsal and phalangeal remnants have been prepared down to vascularized bone as described earlier, we recommend deflating the tourniquet, allowing vascular flow to the hallux, which assists in confirming that the bone ends are vascular; if they are not, additional resection may be required. A laminar spreader is inserted into the defect and slowly distracted until the proposed length of the planned interposition graft has been simulated. If at any point the toe becomes pale or dusky, suggesting dysvascularity, the laminar spreader is slowly released until normal vascular flow to the hallux is reestablished. This length is the maximal length of any interposed graft used in the fusion. If the metatarsal cascade of the lesser metatarsals is not adequately balanced at this point, the surgeon should consider performing a shortening distal oblique sliding osteotomy of the lesser metatarsals to compensate for the difference.

ILIAC CREST TRICORTICAL HARVEST TECHNIQUE

If iliac crest autograft is being harvested, it is recommended that a separate set of instruments be used to decrease the potential risk of cross-contamination and subsequent infection. The incision is made approximately 3 cm proximal to the anterior superior iliac spine in order to avoid injury to the lateral femoral cutaneous nerve, which can result in the painful condition meralgia paresthetica. The size of the incision depends on the size of the graft that is needed, but it is recommended that it should be large enough to allow for adequate visualization. Electrocautery should be used to meticulously dissect down to the periosteum of the iliac crest, which is at the interval between the external oblique and gluteus musculature. The periosteum is initially dissected off the inner and outer tables of the iliac wing and the remainder is bluntly stripped using a Cobb elevator. A sponge can be packed in this region to control any bleeding that may occur. Two large Hohmann retractors are then introduced and the desired segment of bone to be harvested is marked. Using an osteotome or microsagittal saw, the iliac crest is osteotomized to obtain a tricortical bone block. Care must be taken to prevent harvesting a triangular graft by ensuring that the vertical cuts into the crest are parallel. Additional cancellous graft should be obtained so that it can be used to fill any remaining voids in the MTPJ region after the structural graft is secured into the desired position. Per the surgeon's preference, the donor site can be backfilled with either cancellous allograft bone or bone wax and a drain placed, but it is not required. The wound is then closed in layers.

GRAFT FIXATION

The structural graft (either autograft or allograft) should be secured on the back table so that it can be fashioned into the desired shape and size. If a flat-cut technique was performed, a microsagittal saw should be used to make corresponding cuts on the graft so that it aligns the toe in the appropriate position. Again, it is important to irrigate the graft while making the cuts in order to avoid thermal necrosis. If a cup-and-cone reamer was used to prepare the joint, it should also be used to prepare the graft using matching sized reamers. An additional option is to create flat cuts at the metatarsal end of the graft, and a cup-and-cone cut at the distal end of the graft, which allows a stable interface proximally, with an adjustable interface distally, to allow for appropriate positioning of the toe.

If a structural allograft is used, the surgeon can consider harvesting cancellous autograft from the tibia, or the calcaneus to augment the construct. The construct should then be temporarily fixed in the desired position (10° valgus, neutral rotation, 10° dorsiflexion relative to the floor) using Kirschner wires. The positioning is confirmed via simulating weight bearing of the foot using a flat plate (the lid of a surgical tray can be used). The hallux should lie adjacent to, but not touching or overlapping, the second toe, and the distal phalanx should sit 2 to 3 mm off the plate to accommodate an anatomic roll-over during the toe-off phase of gait. If the bone accommodates it, an interfragmentary screw can be placed at this point using either a solid or cannulated screw. A dorsal plate is then applied, ideally under compression at both interfaces. The plate should have options available with which the metatarsal, graft, and phalanx can all be secured through the plate so the risk of graft migration is minimized. An example of plate fixation is shown in **Fig. 5**. After the plate has been fixed into position, a sterile flat plate is used to assess the final position, as shown in **Fig. 6**.

If satisfied with the position, the wound should be irrigated before placing the cancellous autograft, if harvested, into the voids around the construct. The capsule

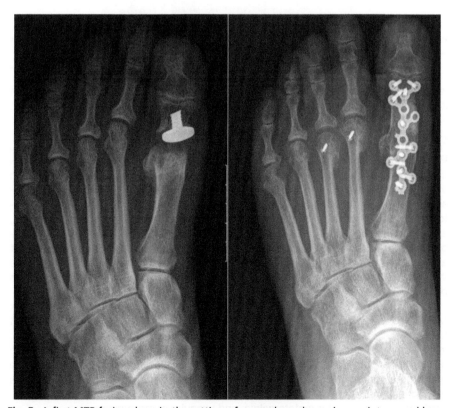

Fig. 5. A first MTP fusion done in the setting of severe bone loss using an interposed bone graft and a plate and screw construct. Second and third metatarsal osteotomies were also added to balance the metatarsal cascade.

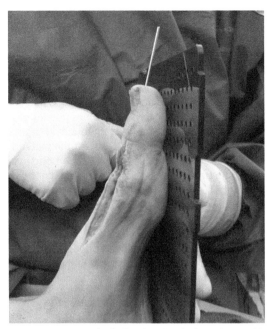

Fig. 6. A key intraoperative step in which the clinician judges the position of the first MTPJ fusion. The flat plate (taken from any sterile set on the operating room table) simulates weight bearing and allows accurate assessment of fusion position intraoperatively.

is then closed over the plate and the EHL tendon repaired at a neutral resting tension if it was lengthened. The subcutaneous tissue and skin are closed in a standard manner.

Complications and Management

Positioning of the toe and MTPJ as described earlier is crucial to obtaining good functional results. The tip of the toe should be able to exert pressure on the ground when the patient is standing and adequately clear the floor when held in a fully extended position. Excessive dorsiflexion of the toe can lead to overload of the sesamoids, symptomatic irritation of the hallux in a shoe, and poor cosmesis. In a similar fashion, excessive plantarflexion can lead to jamming of the distal phalanx during the push-off phase of gait, leading to poor gait mechanics and eventual interphalangeal joint arthrosis. A varus position can make finding comfortable shoe wear difficult because the toe rubs against the shoe, causing pain and ingrown toenails, whereas a valgus position can irritate the second toe.

Nonunion is one of the most common complications of a distraction bone-block MTPJ arthrodesis. This problem often occurs at 1 fusion interface, but can occur at both or either ends of the graft. Nonunion leads to pain and potential hardware failure. In the setting of a nonunion, an external bone stimulator can be used to help promote healing at the graft-host interface, but occasionally revision surgery or addition of bone graft to the nonunion site is required. Other potential complications are the same as exist for a primary MTPJ arthrodesis. These complications include malunion, infection, hardware failure, transfer metatarsalgia, and vascular compromise.

Each of these situations is managed in the same manner as if it were occurring in a primary setting. If infection is ruled out, nonoperative management is limited to rigid orthotics and accommodative shoe wear. If these methods fail to improve the patient's symptoms or infection is present, rerevision surgery is an option but an amputation of the hallux or partial amputation of the first ray can be considered because additional bone loss is to be expected.

Postoperative Care

It is recommended that the patient be non–weight bearing for at least 6 weeks after surgery to allow bone healing either in a cast or a removable boot. Sequential AP, lateral, and oblique radiographs should be obtained to monitor healing at the fusion site and to ensure that the position of the reconstruction remains appropriate. After 6 weeks, progressive weight bearing is permitted in an off-loading boot according to radiographic healing and patient's comfort. When radiographic evidence of union is seen, the patient can be progressed to full weight-bearing status as tolerated in the postoperative shoe, and subsequently into a regular shoe. When using an interposition graft, it usually takes 4 to 6 months to obtain full healing. A graphite shank can be considered to provide the patient with additional support during this transition.

Outcomes

Few outcome studies exist with regard to fusion of the first MTPJ with bone loss/defects. Myerson and colleagues[6] published a retrospective case series on their results using tricortical iliac crest bone graft for restoration of length. Their series included 24 patients (18 women, 6 men) with an average age of 46.4 years. Their indications included prior Silastic arthroplasty, bunionectomy, distal metatarsal osteotomy, Keller resection arthroplasty, and total joint arthroplasty. All subjects had a shortened first metatarsal with associated transfer metatarsalgia, in addition to a painful MTPJ. The bone loss in this case series was associated with osteonecrosis in 9 patients and osteomyelitis in 7 patients. Fourteen patients underwent concurrent procedures that included hammer toe corrections, excision of a Morton neuroma, and lesser metatarsal osteotomies. All patients were evaluated clinically and radiographically at a mean interval of 62.7 months postoperatively. The investigators used the American Orthopaedic Foot and Ankle Society (AOFAS) hallux and MTP 100-point outcome scales. Radiographic and clinical union occurred in 19 of 24 (79%) patients. The 5 nonunions included 2 asymptomatic nonunions and 3 that were revised and ultimately achieved a solid fusion. The mean AOFAS score improved from a mean of 39 points to a mean of 79 points postoperatively. All patients stated that they were satisfied with the procedure and would undergo the surgery again. The investigators concluded that MTP arthrodesis with iliac crest bone graft to restore length was a worthwhile procedure despite the technical difficulties that could be encountered and the high nonunion rate.

A study by Garras and colleagues[11] evaluated clinical outcomes after a conversion arthrodesis for failed first MTPJ hemiarthroplasty. Their study was a retrospective case series in which 18 of the 21 patients were available for follow-up. Preoperative assessment included the visual analogue pain scale (VAS) and the AOFAS Hallux Metatarsophalangeal Interphalangeal (AOFAS-HMI) scoring system. Postoperative outcomes were assessed using the VAS, AOFAS-HMI, and the Foot and Ankle Ability Measure. With regard to surgical technique, 12 cases used local autogenous bone graft and 6 required tricortical iliac crest bone graft for the treatment of extensive bone loss. Final follow-up was at a mean of 4.3 years. Mean VAS pain scores decreased from 7.8 preoperatively to 0.75 postoperatively. Mean AOFAS-HMI improved from 36.2 out of 100 to 85.3 out of 90 (the scale was modified to exclude first MTP motion). All patients achieved union, which was determined radiographically. The investigators concluded that conversion from a failed hallux MTP hemiarthroplasty to an arthrodesis showed similar success to a primary arthrodesis.

Bhosale and colleagues[5] published a retrospective case series examining complex primary arthrodesis of the first MTPJ in the setting of major bone loss. Their series consisted of 10 feet in 9 patients with an average age of 55.9 years and a mean follow-up of 12.6 months. Indications for arthrodesis included 6 failed first MTP total joint arthroplasties and 4 failed Keller resection arthroplasties. This case series assessed patients for satisfaction, pain, clinical/radiographic fusion, and complications. With regard to satisfaction, 8 out of 10 patients were satisfied and pain free at the average time of discharge. Clinical and radiographic union occurred in 9 out of 10 patients. Complications included 1 infection, 2 with prominent hardware, and 1 implant failure. The 1 infection was superficial and this subject did ultimately develop a stable, fibrous union. Overall, the investigators noted that failed arthroplasty (either Keller or total joint) is a difficult problem to manage. Complex primary arthrodesis of the first MTPJ after bone loss was, in their eyes, a viable salvage procedure.

Hecht and colleagues[9] published their retrospective case series that included 16 feet on 14 patients who underwent first MTPJ fusion as a salvage procedure for failed silicone implant arthroplasty. Ten of these needed to be reconstructed with tricortical interposition bone graft because of significant bone loss. Their average duration of follow-up was 55 months, at which time 14 of the 16 had gone on to a solid union (87.5%). They also implemented their own subjective assessment scale, on which scores ranged from 5 (normal) to 0 (severely affected). Pain severity improved from an average of 0.69 preoperatively to 4.89 postoperatively. The average walking tolerance improved from 1.11 to 4.80. The patients' ability to wear shoes improved from 0.87 to 3.1. Overall satisfaction improved from 0.0 to 4.79. The investigators concluded that first MTPJ fusion using bone graft to salvage failed silicone arthroplasties produces acceptable subjective and radiographic results with a high level of patient function and satisfaction.

A systematic review by Mankovecky and colleagues[12] highlighted the challenging nature of performing first MTPJ fusion with autogenous iliac crest bone graft in the setting of a failed Keller arthroplasty. This review documented the incidence of nonunion to be 4.8% (2 out of 42). Their search included 6 studies and included 42 arthrodeses in 40 patients. The mean age was 59 years and the mean follow-up was 42 months. The investigators commented that, despite the revision setting, use of autogenous iliac crest bone graft led to a high rate of union (95.2%).

SUMMARY

First MTPJ joint disorder is a common cause of chronic forefoot pain, deformity, and dysfunction. A wide variety of procedures have been described for this condition that range from resection arthroplasty to total joint arthroplasty and arthrodesis. Failure can produce a significant amount of bone loss in the first MTPJ region. First MTPJ arthrodesis with interpositional bone graft remains the accepted procedure to restore length to the first ray and the foot's normal biomechanics. A general indication to perform a distraction arthrodesis is 1 cm or more of anticipated bone loss and, for this reason, preoperative evaluation is crucial. Tricortical iliac crest is the graft of choice in this situation because it possesses both osteoinductive and osteoconductive properties, but nevertheless it has risks. Although there are few studies in the literature addressing this difficult problem, it seems that, when a solid union is obtained, patients have improved outcome scores, function, and overall satisfaction.

REFERENCES

1. Womack JW, Ishikawa SN. First metatarsophalangeal arthrodesis. Foot Ankle Clin 2009;14(1):43–50.
2. Kumar V, Clough T. Silastic arthroplasty of the first metatarsophalangeal joint as salvage for failed revisional fusion with interpositional structural bone graft. BMJ Case Rep 2013;2013 [pii:bcr2013008993].
3. Gibson JN, Thomson CE. Arthrodesis or total replacement arthroplasty for hallux rigidus: a randomized controlled trial. Foot Ankle Int 2005;26(9):680–90.
4. Pulavarti RS, McVie JL, Tulloch CJ. First metatarsophalangeal joint replacement using the bio-action great toe implant: intermediate results. Foot Ankle Int 2005;26(12):1033–7.
5. Bhosale A, Munoruth A, Blundell C, et al. Complex primary arthrodesis of the first metatarsophalangeal joint after bone loss. Foot Ankle Int 2011;32(10):968–72.
6. Myerson MS, Schon LC, McGuigan FX, et al. Result of arthrodesis of the hallux metatarsophalangeal joint using bone graft for restoration of length. Foot Ankle Int 2000;21(4):297–306.
7. Bennett GL, Kay DB, Sabatta J. First metatarsophalangeal joint arthrodesis: an evaluation of hardware failure. Foot Ankle Int 2005;26(8):593–6.
8. Whalen JL. Clinical tip: interpositional bone graft for first MP fusion. Foot Ankle Int 2009;30(2):160–2.
9. Hecht PJ, Gibbons MJ, Wapner KL, et al. Arthrodesis of the first metatarsophalangeal joint to salvage failed silicone implant arthroplasty. Foot Ankle Int 1997;18(7): 383–90.
10. Schuh R, Trnka HJ. First metatarsophalangeal arthrodesis for severe bone loss. Foot Ankle Clin 2011;16(1):13–20.
11. Garras DN, Durinka JB, Bercik M, et al. Conversion arthrodesis for failed first metatarsophalangeal joint hemiarthroplasty. Foot Ankle Int 2013;34(9):1227–32.
12. Mankovecky MR, Prissel MA, Roukis TS. Incidence of nonunion of first metatarsophalangeal joint arthrodesis with autogenous iliac crest bone graft after failed Keller-Brandes arthroplasty: a systematic review. J Foot Ankle Surg 2013;52(1): 53–5.

The Use of Osteotomy in the Management of Hallux Rigidus

 CrossMark

Raheel Shariff, FRCS (Tr & Orth)[a],*, Mark S. Myerson, MD[b]

KEYWORDS

- Functional hallux rigidus • Osteotomies for hallux rigidus • Osteotomy
- Metatarsalphalangeal joint

KEY POINTS

- Metatarsus elevatus and gastrocnemius tightness contribute to the development of functional hallux rigidus.
- Although several osteotomies have been described for functional hallux rigidus, certain osteotomies are commonly used in practice for the correction of functional hallux rigidus, a long first metatarsal or an elevated metatarsal, or an unstable tarsometatarsal (TMT) joint.
- Proximal plantarflexion osteotomy is used only in the presence of an elevated first metatarsal with a limit to dorsiflexion but without the presence of arthritis at the first metatarsophalangeal (MP) joint.
- In the presence of arthritis at the MP joint, the decision is between an oblique distal metatarsal osteotomy (the authors prefer the Maceira type) and the shortening periarticular osteotomy.

INTRODUCTION

Hallux rigidus is a condition characterized by degenerative changes to the first MP joint. It is the second most common condition to affect the first MP joint after hallux valgus and the most frequently occurring degenerative condition in the foot. The condition was first described by Davies-Colley[1] in 1887; however, it was Cotterill[2] who coined the term, *hallux rigidus.*

The exact etiology of this condition is not well understood, although several factors have been put forth as contributing causes. Trauma, osteochondral lesions,[3] inflammatory arthropathies, including gout, rheumatoid arthritis, and seronegative arthropathies, have all been said to contribute to this condition. Biomechanical and

The authors have nothing to disclose.
[a] Trauma and Orthopaedic Surgery, Central Manchester University Hospitals - NHS Foundation Trust, Oxford Road, Manchester, UK; [b] The Institute for Foot and Ankle Reconstruction at Mercy Medical Centre, 301 St Paul Pl, Baltimore, MD 21202, USA
* Corresponding author.
E-mail address: shariffstays@gmail.com

structural factors are also believed to play a part. Lambrinudi[4] suggested that an elevated first ray contributes to flexion at the hallux IP joint.[4,5] Pronation, hallux valgus interphalangeus, hallux valgus, and hypermobility of the first ray have all been implicated.[6,7] None of these theories, however, has been proved and only Coughlin[5] has shown a correlation between hallux valgus interphalangeus and hallux rigidus. It is possible that metatarsus elevatus and gastrocnemius tightness contribute to the development of functional hallux rigidus; their role is further delineated in this article. There are several osteotomies that have been described in the literature, but the authors focus on those they commonly use for correction of functional hallux rigidus, a long first metatarsal or an elevated metatarsal, or an unstable TMT joint.

CLASSIFICATION

Several classification systems have been described for this condition. The Hattrupp and Johnson[8] classification system examines the degree of osteophyte formation and amount of joint space narrowing on radiographs but is not validated. The Coughlin and Shurnas classification is a comprehensive clinical and radiographic grading that differs from other systems in that it has a grade 4 characterized by pain in the mid-range of movement.[9] Although classification systems may be useful for descriptive purposes in the evaluation and treatment of hallux rigidus, the authors believe that hallux rigidus may be functional or structural, and this is a far simpler approach to the problem. Functional hallux rigidus is characterized by good passive dorsiflexion at the first MP joint when the patient is not weight bearing but reduced passive dorsiflexion when the foot is loaded and the patient is weight bearing.[10,11] In other words, there is good dorsiflexion in open chain movements but reduced in closed chain movements. It is unlikely that all cases of structural hallux rigidus begin as a form of structural hallux rigidus, but it is clear that the latter is a more advanced form of the same spectrum wherein passive dorsiflexion is reduced even during non–weight-bearing conditions. It is crucial to understand that examination of the first MP joint under non–weight-bearing conditions does not give information regarding its behavior during gait.[12,13]

If there is good range of movement during non–weight-bearing examination, it should be possible to improve pain and in all likelihood improve the movement during weight bearing by osteotomies and other joint-preserving procedures. On the other hand, if there is first metatarsal joint jamming during dorsiflexion or an elevated or long first metatarsal, this condition may also benefit from an osteotomy even if there is decreased range of movement when the joint is not loaded. If there is little movement in non–weight-bearing conditions (in the absence of the conditions discussed previously), the authors believe that arthrodesis or arthoplasty procedures are the preferred choice, irrespective of what the radiologic findings are. This is why differentiating between functional and structural hallux rigidus is crucial and a good working classification.

PATHOLOGY

The functional inter-relationship between the triceps surae and the plantar arch was first described by Arandes and Viladot in 1956. They described the Achilles-calcaneal plantar plate system based on the work of Seiberg in 1936. They suggested that the bony intermediate position of this system, the calcaneal tuberosity, is akin to a large sesamoid bone and transmits the flexor power of the triceps surae to the forefoot (Arandes and Viladot). The organ of the heel is the archetypical fibrocartilaginous enthesis model and guarantees functional continuity between the Achilles and the calcaneal plantar plate system. Weight-bearing range of motion at the first MP joint is dependent on structures that are based more proximally, specifically the Achilles-calcaneal plantar system. A tight gastrocsoleus complex blocks ankle dorsiflexion during the progression from the second to third rocker of gait. A restriction to ankle passive dorsiflexion increases dorsiflexion moments at the forefoot, thus increasing tensile stress at the plantar soft tissues due to the truss and beam mechanism of the plantar vault support. A failure to achieve first metatarsal plantar flexion or an increased tensile stress through the plantar fascia limits passive dorsiflexion at the first MP joint during its transition from the second to third rocker. Limited passive dorsiflexion of the first MP joint blocks motion in the sagittal plane, which is necessary for the forward progression of the body during gait and also produces a rolling contact at the dorsal portion of the first MP joint as opposed to gliding contact. The latter further contributes to development of degenerative changes within the joint.

Compensatory mechanisms must develop to cope with the lack of motion at the first MP joint. They may or may not lead to the onset of symptoms. An elevated position of the head of the first metatarsal with respect to the proximal phalanx or an increase in tension in the plantar aponeurosis also induces a tendency toward rolling contact pattern in the first MP joint during the transition from the second to the third rocker. It is debatable whether the elevation of the head of the first metatarsal is the primary mechanical anomaly or whether the increase in tension in the plantar aponeurosis is the culprit. Regardless of which comes first, an alteration in the opposite occurs (ie the windlass tightening or elevation of the first metatarsal). This alteration in gait pattern (described previously) alters the motion at the first MP joint from a gliding to a rolling movement within the joint, with an inherent block to dorsiflexion. This progressively leads to degenerative changes due to abnormal joint kinematics.

DIAGNOSIS OF FUNCTIONAL HALLUX RIGIDUS

Patients complain of pain overlying the first MP joint and difficulty with toe off. There may be a dorsal osteophyte present and synovitis due to irritation of the medial dorsal branch of the superficial peroneal nerve due to the osteophytes. The range of motion of the first MP joint should be assessed in the non–weight-bearing and weight-bearing conditions, ideally with patients supine. Simulated weight bearing is performed by pushing on the first metatarsal upwards until the ankle is in a neutral position. The proximal phalanx is then grasped and passively dorsiflexed. If the hallux MP joint has adequate function, there is approximately 90° of dorsiflexion at the first MP joint in this position or at least greater than 60°. The test is considered positive and patients considered to have functional hallux rigidus if the ankle moves on dorsiflexing the proximal phalanx and not the first MP joint. The authors consider that a diagnosis of functional hallux rigidus cannot be established if 60° of dorsiflexion is exceeded on performing the test. Other associated conditions, such as a pronated foot and plantar callosities due to transfer metatarsalgia, should also be looked for.

MANAGEMENT

The authors are not in favor of surgical intervention for the nonsymptomatic functional hallux rigidus. Usually such patients present to a clinic due to decreased range of motion at the first metatarsal joint and absence of any pain. This is because results are unpredictable and surgery should be undertaken only once a patient complains of a mechanical block or pain. Nonoperative intervention may be tried in the form of modification of footwear and orthosis. The use of a rocker bottom sole compensates for the alterations in the second rocker (ankle block) and third rocker (first MP joint block).

Response to this type of footwear is variable, however, and forefoot pronation should be taken into account when prescribing orthotic supports.

SURGICAL MANAGEMENT

The contribution of the gastrocnemius to the pathogenesis of this condition is common, and, if a gastrocnemius contracture is present, then partial selective lengthening of the triceps surae complex is undertaken as part of the surgical algorithm. On confirming that a patient has preserved movement at the first MP joint when the first ray is not loaded (non–weight bearing), then osteotomies can safely be performed to modify the arc of movement such that the range of motion improves during weight bearing. As a general principle, the authors are opposed to an angular osteotomy proximally in the metatarsal. This is because in hallux rigidus the authors find that degenerative changes are usually found in the dorsal third of the metatarsal head. If a proximally based plantar flexion osteotomy is performed, this makes the abnormal dorsal portion of the metatarsal head to articulate more, and not less, with the proximal phalanx as the metatarsal head has been rotated in a plantarward direction. In cases of a true metatarsus elevatus with functional hallux rigidus, where there is none or limited articular erosion, however, a proximal angular osteotomy is an acceptable procedure to perform.

DISTAL METATARSAL OSTEOTOMIES

Several metatarsal osteotomies have been described for hallux rigidus in literature. The function of any of these osteotomies is to decompress the joint by shortening the first metatarsal, correct functional hallux rigidus secondary to metatarsus primus elevatus by plantar flexing the first ray, or realign the joint surface to create a more functional arc of movement. Although there are numerous osteotomies described in the literature, the authors restrict this presentation to those they use regularly.

Watermann-Green Osteotomy

Most of these osteotomy procedures commence with a dorsal cheilectomy as needed. In some cases of pure functional hallux rigidus, this is be necessary because the articular surface in the nonloaded position is essentially normal. This is a 2-arm chevron-type osteotomy using a medial longitudinal approach over the first metatarsal.[14] The dorsal arm consists of 2 incomplete osteotomies, approximately 1 cm proximal to the articular surface of the metatarsal head. This enables a slice of bone to be removed, thereby shortening the first metatarsal and decompressing the joint. The slice of bone can be cut in many different ways, for example, as a wedge that can thereby change the metatarsal articular angle. The second arm of the osteotomy is the plantar arm that was originally described to be at 135° to the dorsal arm. This osteotomy can be modified, however, such that if a trapezoidal wedge is removed from the incomplete dorsal arm, the articular surface can be realigned.[15] Also the angle of the plantar arm can be altered to change the ratio of the metatarsal shortening to the plantar displacement of the head.

The authors' indication for this osteotomy is the presence of functional hallux rigidus due to an elongated first ray with the presence of dorsal articular erosion but preserved articular surface plantarly, because this procedure enables realigning this healthy cartilage to articulate with the proximal phalanx as well as shorten the metatarsal. It is contraindicated if there is no preserved articular cartilage plantarly even if shortening with the dorsal wedge decompresses the joint, because, in the authors' experience, patients continue to remain symptomatic. Given the versatility of this osteotomy and the variables that can be altered, it should be used with caution, because one of the side effects could be overzealous plantar displacement of the distal metatarsal head fragment, which could give rise to increase stresses on the metatarsosesamoid joint. This in turn could cause sesamoiditis and first metatarsalgia. Retrospective studies have shown good results with this procedure. Dickerson and colleagues[16] reported retrospectively on 28 patients; 94% reported significant relief of pain and 75% had a subjective improvement in range of motion at a mean 4-year follow-up.

The Authors' Preferred Technique: Youngswick Osteotomy

The Youngswick osteotomy is a stable osteotomy[17] and easy to perform and it is easy to control the amount of shortening of the first metatarsal. It is indicated in particular with a long first metatarsal to accomplish slight shortening and lowering of the head. The authors also use this osteotomy for correction of hallux valgus associated with functional hallux rigidus where some shortening of the metatarsal in addition to the lateral shift of the head is beneficial.

It is a V-shaped chevron osteotomy with the apex based distally. The chevron cuts are made at a 60° angle, and then a third cut is made parallel to the dorsal arm of the osteotomy to take out a sliver of bone and enable shortening of the metatarsal. This helps decompress the MP joint. It also aims to slightly lower the metatarsal head as it is decompressed to reduce dorsal impingement.

Ollof and colleagues retrospectively reviewed the results of this procedure in 28 patients for advanced hallux rigidus. At 5.7-year follow-up, they found 85% of patients reporting satisfactory outcomes, with 75% of these patients claiming more than 90% improvement in symptoms. No objective outcomes or scoring systems, however, were used in this study.[18] The investigators also combined adjunctive procedures, such as chondroplasty and cheilectomies, without specifying the numbers of these adjunctive procedures, thereby making it difficult to draw strong conclusions. Giannini and colleagues[19] reviewed a series of 8 patients who underwent this procedure for severe hallux rigidus and found an improvement in American Orthopaedic Foot and Ankle Society (AOFAS) scores and range of movement at the first MP joint.

The main concern the authors have with this procedure is the risk of avascular necrosis and shortening of the first metatarsal, which may contribute to transfer metatarsalgia. Because shortening is inevitable and, as described previously, even desirable in the presence of a long first ray, plantar translation usually compensates for it and prevents any transfer metatarsalgia.

This osteotomy differs from the Waterman-Green osteotomy. The principal difference is the angle between the plantar and dorsal limbs, which is more acute with the Youngswick type (60°) versus the Watermann-Green type (135°). It is difficult to differentiate between these 2 procedures in practice because there is a lot of overlap between them. They are both versatile osteotomies and the angle between these 2 can be variable depending on whether shortening or plantar displacement is more necessary, making it hard to differentiate one from the other.

The authors prefer the Youngswick osteotomy for a variety of reasons. Given that the angle is acute between the plantar and dorsal limbs compared with the Watermann – Green type, it facilitates a longer plantar limb to the osteotomy, making it inherently more stable and easier to fix with a screw. It also has a greater surface area of contact for union. The limitation with this osteotomy is that because the angle between the 2 limbs is acute, the degree of plantar displacement that can be achieved is restricted; however, the balance between stability and degree of plantar displacement needs to be determined when performing this osteotomy. A study looking at this osteotomy in 23 feet at 2-year follow-up noted an increase by 28% in peak pressures under the first metatarsal head due to the plantar displacement. What this means clinically, however, particularly with regard to sesamoid symptoms, is not clear in literature.[20] **Fig. 1** illustrates this osteotomy.

The authors' indication for this osteotomy is functional hallux rigidus with an elongated first metatarsal, which requires shortening and plantarflexion of the head, particularly in the presence of hallux valgus.

OBLIQUE DISTAL METATARSAL OSTEOTOMY

This osteotomy was first described by Lundeen[21] for the treatment of hallux valgus, which was associated with hallux rigidus; however, it is predominantly used for hallux rigidus. It consists of an oblique osteotomy made from a dorsal distal to plantar proximal direction angled at approximately 30° to the sagittal plane. The metatarsal head is then displaced proximally and plantar ward, thereby decompressing the first MP joint and plantar displacement of the head.

Malerba and colleagues[22] reported retrospectively on 20 patients with an 11-year follow-up after this procedure. They concluded that this was a safe reliable procedure based on high AOFAS scores and improved range of movement. Several other retrospective studies have reported satisfactory results with this technique although no definite statistical analysis was performed in most of these studies.[6,19,23,24] None of them reported significant complications, such as avascular necrosis of the head or nonunion at the osteotomy site. **Fig. 2** delineates this osteotomy.

The Authors' Preferred Indications and Technique

The authors use this type of osteotomy where an elongated first metatarsal is the only contributing pathology. They do not tend to use it in cases of an elevated metatarsal because in the latter condition, a distal shortening chevron-type procedure is beneficial to realign the articular surface, as described previously.

A dorsal longitudinal incision over the first MP joint is made and the EHL is retracted laterally. The metatarsal head is exposed and, with the proximal phalanx placed in flexion, a minimal cheilectomy is performed. The first cut is at a 30° angle to the first metatarsal, commencing just above the articular surface. The desired

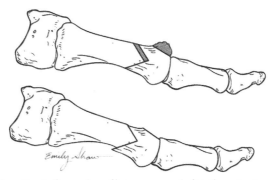

Fig. 1. The shaded portion is the wedge of bone removed after the osteotomy in the metatarsal shown in *upper* figure and associated dorsal cheilectomy. Note the plantar displacement achieved shown in *lower* part of figure. (*Courtesy of* Mark S. Myerson, MD, Mercy Medical Centre, Baltimore, MD, USA)

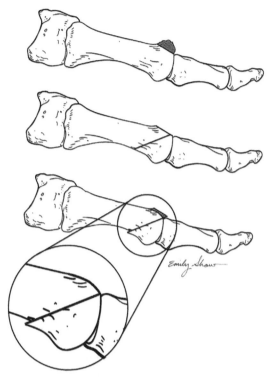

Fig. 2. Oblique distal osteotomy used for an elongated first metatarsal head shown in *middle* and *lower* part of the figure. The *topmost* part of the figure shows the cheilectomy. (*Courtesy of* Mark S. Myerson, MD, Mercy Medical Centre, Baltimore, MD, USA)

amount of metatarsal shortening is templated and determined preoperatively on the radiographs. The second cut is then made vertically from dorsal to plantar, approximately 4 to 5 mm proximal to the apex of the first osteotomy. This is an incomplete cut and is stopped as soon as the plantar fragment is reached. The third cut then involves removing a small sliver of bone from the distal metatarsal and then the head is shortened and slightly angulated dorsally so that there is articular cartilage and not bone on the dorsal articular surface. This maneuver is advantageous because it is precise and the amount of shortening is able to be controlled, depending on how far proximal the second cut is made. This is because proximal translation of the head is done just up to the level of where the second vertical cut was made, thereby enabling determining the shortening. It also maintains articular contact throughout the range of motion and eliminates the pathologic dorsal rim of the joint. **Fig. 3** explains the cuts in this osteotomy.

PROXIMAL METATARSAL OSTEOTOMY

A simple plantar flexion osteotomy of the proximal aspect of the metatarsal works best in the authors' experience. As discussed previously, however, care should be taken to ensure that there is no arthritis at the first MP joint when using this procedure. If there is any evidence of arthritis, then a distal osteotomy is performed. The authors' indication for a proximal plantarflexion osteotomy of the metatarsal is the presence of functional

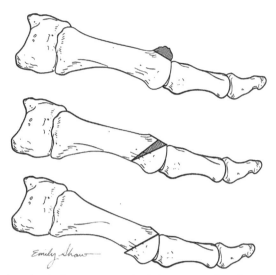

Fig. 3. The shaded wedge is the portion excised. (*Courtesy of* Mark S. Myerson, MD, Mercy Medical Centre, Baltimore, MD, USA)

hallux rigidus with gross elevation of the first metatarsal, limited dorsiflexion of the first MP joint, and no arthritis at the MP joint. The principle of this osteotomy is to reduce intrinsic contracture present as a result of first metatarsal elevation. The short flexors contract and gliding of the volar plate apparatus is restricted. With a plantar closing wedge osteotomy, the relaxation that occurs in the plantar musculature and ligaments improves motion.

A medial longitudinal incision over the proximal aspect of the first metatarsal is made. After subperiosteal dissection and soft tissue retraction, the entire base of the metatarsal is visible. A plantar-based wedge is removed approximately 5 mm wide at the base of the wedge. The dorsal cortex is kept intact to facilitate closure of the osteotomy. Once the wedge is removed, the hallux is dorsiflexed and, while this maneuver is performed, pressure is exerted onto the metatarsal head and the distal metatarsal is pushed down into plantar flexion, facilitating a closure of the osteotomy. A 2-hole plantar locking plate is then used to fix this osteotomy (**Fig. 4**).

MODIFIED LAPIDUS PROCEDURE

In the presence of significant first TMT joint instability with elevation of the metatarsal, the modified Lapidus procedure is the option of choice for the authors. Care must be taken to use this procedure only in the presence of significant first TMT joint instability.

A dorsal incision is made to approach the TMT joint. After subperiosteal dissection, care is taken to denude only the articular cartilage from either side of the joint surfaces. A laminar spreader is used to distract the joint and gain access to the plantar side of the joint where thorough preparation of the joint surface should be performed. The key with this procedure is to dial in the plantarflexion of the first metatarsal prior to fixation. This is performed with a maneuver similar to the one described previously with hyperdorsiflexion of the hallux, which plantarflexes the

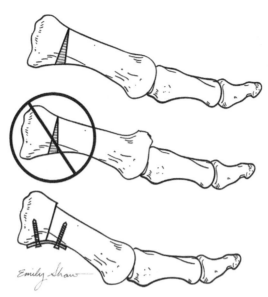

Fig. 4. Note that once a plantar-based wedge of bone is taken, the metatarsal is also displaced slightly plantarwards. (*Courtesy of* Mark S. Myerson, MD, Mercy Medical Centre, Baltimore, MD, USA)

metatarsal and the osteotomy is then fixed with 2 screws across the joint, diagonally crossing each other.

SUMMARY

The literature is replete with several types of osteotomies that aim to relieve symptoms secondary to hallux rigidus. The problem with these osteotomies is that current evidence is poor because the procedures performed are heterogeneous in the studies performed, often with a combination of an osteotomy with a cheilectomy, which confounds the results. Also the studies are not robust and good-quality clinical trials are lacking to draw strong conclusions. The other problem is that most of the osteotomies discussed previously are based on a presumption of a causal relationship between hallux elevates or a long first metatarsal and hallux rigidus, although there is no definite proof that this is the case.

The authors, believe, however, that such a relationship exists. Their treatment algorithm is to use a proximal plantarflexion osteotomy only in the presence of an elevated first metatarsal with a limit to dorsiflexion but without the presence of arthritis at the first MP joint. In the presence of arthritis at the MP joint, the decision is between an oblique distal metatarsal osteotomy (the authors prefer the Maceira type) and the shortening periarticular osteotomy (the authors prefer a shortening chevron type similar to a Youngswick osteotomy). In the presence of arthritis with just an elongated first metatarsal, a Maceira-type osteotomy is the preferred option. But if the aim is to shorten and plantarflex the metatarsal head, a periarticular osteotomy, such as a shortening chevron type, is the authors' chosen option.

These procedures associated with a dorsal cheilectomy involving a third of the dorsal articular cartilage of the first metatarsal head in patients with functional hallux rigidus even in the presence of significant radiographic changes are successful, the key being to select the right patient profile.

REFERENCES

1. Davies-Colley M. Contraction of the metatarso-phalangeal joint of the great toe. BMJ 1887;1:728.
2. Cotteril JM. Stiffness of the great toe in adolescents. British Med J 1888;1:158.
3. Nilsonne H. Hallux rigidus and its treatment. Acta Orthop Scand 1930;1:295–303.
4. Lambrinudi P. Metatarsus primus elevatus. Proc R Soc Med 1938;31:1273.
5. Coughlin MJ, Shurnas PS. Hallux rigidus: demographics, etiology, and radiographic assessment. Foot Ankle Int 2003;24(10):731–43.
6. Drago J, Oloff L, Jacobs AM. A comprehensive review of hallux limitus. J Foot Surg 1984;23(3):213–20.
7. Hattrup SJ, Johnson KA. Subjective results of hallux rigidus following treatment with cheilectomy. Clin Orthop Related Res 1988;226:182–91.
8. Coughlin MJ, Shurnas PS. Hallux rigidus: grading and long-term results of operative treatment. J Bone Joint Surg Am 2003;85(11):2072–88.
9. Roukis TS. Metatarsus primus elevatus in hallux rigidus. Fact or fiction? J Am Podiatr Med Assoc 2005;95(3):221–8.
10. Dananberg HJ. Functional hallux limitus and its relationship to gait efficiency. J Am Podiatr Med Assoc 1986;76(12):648–52.
11. Roukis TS, Scherer PR, Anderson CF. Position of the first ray and motion of the first metatarsophalangeal joint. J Am Podiatr Med Assoc 1996;86:538.
12. Kirby KA. Foot and lower extremity biomechanics II: Precision Intricast Newsletters, 1997-2002. Payson (AZ): Precision Intricast Inc; 2002.
13. Cavolo DJ, Cavallaro DC, Arrington LE, et al. The Watermann osteotomy for hallux limitus. J Am Podiatry Assoc 1979;69:52–7.
14. Laakmann G, Green R, Green D. The modified watermann procedure: a preliminary retrospective study. Podiatry Institute; 1996. Updates. Available at: https://www.podiatryinstitute.com/pdfs/Update_2001/2001_07.pdf.
15. Dickerson JB, Green R, Green DR. Long-term follow-up of the Green-Watermann osteotomy for hallux limitus. J Am Podiatr Med Assoc 2002;92:543–54.
16. Youngswick FD. Modifications of the Austin bunionectomy for treatment of metatarsus primus elevates associated with hallux limitus. J Foot Surg 1982;21:114–6.
17. Oloff LM, Jhala-Patel G. A retrospective analysis of joint sal- vage procedures for grades III and IV hallux rigidus. J Foot Ankle Surg 2008;47:230–6.
18. Giannini S, Ceccarelli F, Faldini C, et al. What's new in surgical options for hallux rigi- dus? J Bone Joint Surg Am 2004;86-A(Suppl 2):2–83.
19. Bryant AR, Tinley P, Cole JH. Plantar pressure and joint mo- tion after the Youngswick procedure for hallux limitus. J Am Podiatr Med Assoc 2004;94:22–30.
20. Lundeen RO, Rose JM. Sliding oblique osteotomy for the treatment of hallux abducto valgus associated with function- al hallux limitus. J Foot Ankle Surg 2000;39:161–7.
21. Malerba F, Milani R, Sartorelli E, et al. Distal oblique first metatarsal osteotomy in grade 3 hallux rigidus: a long- term followup. Foot Ankle Int 2008;29:677–82.
22. Ronconi P, Monachino P, Baleanu PM, et al. Distal oblique osteotomy of the first metatarsal for the correction of hallux lim- itus and rigidus deformity. J Foot Ankle Surg 2000;39:154–60.
23. Gonzalez JV, Garrett PP, Jordan MJ, et al. The modified Hohmann osteotomy: an alternative joint salvage pro- cedure for hallux rigidus. J Foot Ankle Surg 2004;43:380–8.
24. Myerson MS. Reconstructive foot & ankle surgery: management of complications. 2nd edition. Elseiver Saunders; 2010.

Proximal Phalanx Hemiarthroplasty for the Treatment of Advanced Hallux Rigidus

Connor Delman, BS[a], Chris Kreulen, MD[a],
Martin Sullivan, MD, FRACS[b], Eric Giza, MD[a],*

KEYWORDS

* MTP joint * Hallux rigidus * Arthroplasty * Arthrodesis

KEY POINTS

* Multiple treatment options exist for the management of late-stage hallux rigidus.
* The goals of treatment are pain reduction and restoration of function.
* Arthrodesis remains the treatment of choice, but recent advances support the use of first metatarsophalangeal (MTP) hemiarthroplasty as a viable and successful option in properly selected patients in whom preservation of motion and function are desirable.

INTRODUCTION

Hallux rigidus is the most common arthritic condition of the foot and the second most prevalent pathologic condition affecting the big toe.[1,2] It is an osteoarthritic process caused by the progressive destruction of cartilage at the articulation of the first MTP joint, a reduction in the articular space, subchondral sclerosis, subchondral cysts, and osteophyte formation.[3,4] This degenerative process begins dorsally with osteophyte formation that can lead to decreased range of motion.[1] It is often bilateral and idiopathic but may occasionally be associated with prior trauma.[4,5] Loss of motion at the MTP joint of the great toe can lead to adaptive processes such as eversion of the foot and load transfer to the outer border of the foot.[6] Hallux rigidus is more common in

Dr Giza is a consultant for Arthrex and Zimmer, and he has received fellowship funding from Arthrex, and a research grant from Zimmer. Dr Kreulen is a consultant for Arthrex. Drs Delman and Sullivan have nothing to disclose.
[a] Department of Orthopaedics, University of California, Davis, 4860 Y Street, Suite 3800, Sacramento, CA 95817, USA; [b] Foot & Ankle Clinic, St. Vincents Clinic, Suite 901E, 438 Victoria Street Darlinghurst, Sydney, Australia
* Corresponding author.
E-mail address: egiza@ucdavis.edu

Foot Ankle Clin N Am 20 (2015) 503–512
http://dx.doi.org/10.1016/j.fcl.2015.05.002
1083-7515/15/$ – see front matter © 2015 Elsevier Inc. All rights reserved.

foot.theclinics.com

women, primarily affects older individuals, and is associated with hallux valgus inter-phalangeus.[2,4] With an aging population, an increase in the prevalence of this condition is expected.[1]

The treatment options for hallux rigidus depend on the severity of first MTP joint arthritis. Surgical intervention is reserved for patients who fail conservative treatment. The most widely used classification system for determining the grade of hallux rigidus is that described by Coughlin and Shurnas.[7] Nonoperative treatment includes shoe and activity modification, physical therapy, and nonsteroidal anti-inflammatory medications.[8] Intra-articular steroid injections are also used to relieve painful symptoms. Failure of nonoperative treatments may lead to the recommendation for surgery.[4,5,9,10]

Cheilectomy or metatarsal/phalangeal osteotomy is recommended for the initial stages of the disease (grades I and II); however, these procedures are less successful in advanced disease (grades III and IV).[4,11–17] Surgical options for more severe hallux rigidus (grades III and IV) include MTP joint arthroplasty, arthrodesis, soft-tissue arthroplasty, and excisional arthroplasty.[2,5,18–25] Although these procedures can be successful in select cases, each procedure has its limitations and complications.

The Keller excisional arthroplasty has a simple postoperative recovery and is less invasive than arthrodesis, but the procedure can lead to transfer metatarsalgia, cock-up toe deformity, claw toe, valgus drift, and a shortened first ray. It is thus recommended for low-demand, elderly patients or as a salvage procedure.[16,26,27]

Arthrodesis is considered an accepted treatment advanced stages of hallux rigidus.[10,14,16,28] Despite this, there are some disadvantages and potential complications associated with the procedure. These include nonunion, malalignment, stress placed on the adjacent joint, limitation of recreational activities, shoe wearing difficulty, and long recovery periods.[17,21,26,29–33] Range of motion loss may be poorly tolerated by young, active patients and may impair recreational activities.[34]

MTP arthroplasty, which is a joint-preserving procedure, can beneficially restore joint motion. However, potential risks include malposition, implant fracture, stress fracture, arthrofibrosis, and synovitis, all of which can lead to failure.[5,35–37] Silastic and metal-on-polyethylene implant failure can lead to bone loss and shortening, creating difficult salvage procedures.[22,35,37]

During the treatment of hallux rigidus, care must be taken to maintain the stability and function of the MTP joint. The insertion of the plantar aponeurosis into the proximal phalanx and the balance of hallux flexor-extensor and abductor-adductor mechanisms are critical for preserving joint stability.[18,38] The first MTP joint is also subject to compressive loads from associated muscle action.[18] Furthermore, dorsal gliding of the proximal phalanx on the metatarsal head dissipates shear stress during gait, making it an ideal candidate for hemiarthroplasty.[17,39] Arthroplasty procedures that replace the metatarsal head are susceptible to both shear and compressive stresses, which can ultimately lead to prosthetic loosening and failure.[17,18] In contrast, first phalangeal hemiarthroplasty maintains a favorable mechanical arrangement owing to the dorsal gliding of the proximal phalanx on the metatarsal head with weight bearing. The weight bearing characteristics are unlikely to change appreciably after the procedure, reducing the risk of transfer metatarsalgia. Additional advantages include the maintenance of toe length and sesamoid attachments to the proximal phalanx and minimal bone-stock resection.[17,40]

The Arthrex AnaToemic Phalangeal Prosthesis (Arthrex, Inc, Naples, FL, USA) allows for the resurfacing of the base of the proximal phalanx (**Fig. 1**). The small size of the implant requires minimal bone resection, which allows retention of the flexor attachment.[41]

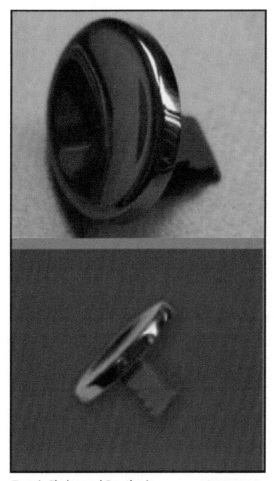

Fig. 1. Arthrex AnaToemic Phalangeal Prosthesis.

INDICATIONS

First MTP hemiarthroplasty is indicated in patients with grade III or IV hallux rigidus who have failed at least 6 months to 1 year of conservative treatment. It is ideal for the low-demand, less active patient older than 65 years. These patients are at lower risk of failure because of diminished forces acting on the surgical implant.[42] This procedure should be done only in patients with a well-aligned and stable first MTP joint.

CONTRAINDICATIONS

Hemiarthroplasty is not recommended in young, highly active patients because of an increased risk of failure.[42] Other contraindications include hallux valgus, inflammatory arthropathy, sesamoid MTP arthritis, previous MTP infection, failed MTP fusion, and impaired peripheral circulation.

PREOPERATIVE PLANNING

The diagnosis of hallux rigidus is confirmed by a thorough history, clinical examination, and radiographic findings. Patients present with a complaint of pain localized to the dorsal first MTP joint with weight bearing. The pain is often worsened in bare feet or when wearing either soft-soled or high-heeled shoes. Symptoms are frequently associated with heavy labor or activities that require extension of the first MTP joint such as walking up stairs, squatting, and running. Patients may also experience lateral metatarsalgia due to alterations in gait and overload of the lateral border of the foot to avoid dorsiflexion through the painful joint.[41,43] The hallux sesamoid joint must be carefully evaluated to exclude it as the source of pain. Physical findings include increased joint size, everted gait, restricted joint motion, and palpable osteophytes on the dorsal aspect of the first metatarsal head. There is also limited dorsiflexion and pain with joint motion that may be associated with crepitus.[2,43]

Imaging should include weight-bearing anteroposterior, lateral, and oblique radiographs (**Fig. 2**). Sesamoid views should be taken if the patient has plantar first MTP pain or tenderness (**Fig. 3**). Severity is graded according to the Coughlin and Shurnas radiographic classification system.[14] Radiographic findings include osteophyte formation, subchondral sclerosis, joint space narrowing, and alteration of the metatarsal head.[2]

OPERATIVE TECHNIQUE

The procedure is performed with the patient in the supine position and under general anesthesia, using a thigh tourniquet or with an ankle block using a pediatric ankle tourniquet. The first MTP joint is exposed through a dorsal longitudinal incision followed by an eccentrically placed longitudinal capsular incision. The capsule is released with preservation of the collateral ligaments and plantar capsule.

Dorsal osteophytes are removed from the proximal phalanx and dorsal metatarsal head, and the medial prominence of the metatarsal head is resected. About 20% to 30% of the articular surface can be resected and is often needed to achieve adequate

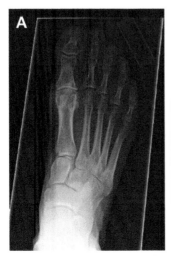
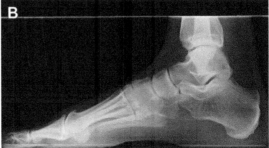

Fig. 2. Anteroposterior (*A*) and lateral (*B*) radiographs of a 67-year-old man with grade III hallux rigidus looking to improve range of motion to continue wearing ski boots.

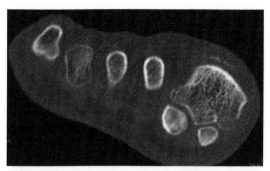

Fig. 3. Axial computed tomographic image demonstrating minimal sesamoid metatarsal osteoarthritis.

postoperative dorsiflexion. A Freer elevator is placed under the metatarsal head to release plantar adhesions. A cut is made perpendicular to the long axis of the proximal phalanx, resecting an amount of bone corresponding to the width of the implant (2.4 mm) (**Fig. 4**).

A centralizing hole is drilled, and a small Hoke osteotome is used to create medial and lateral keel entry points, following which the keel punch is placed into the proximal phalanx (**Fig. 5**). A trial implant is placed to check size, fit, and range of motion. The final implant is then inserted with thumb pressure and carefully seated with an impactor (**Fig. 6**).

The medial capsule is reefed if necessary, and the dorsal capsule is closed with absorbable suture. Range of motion is checked, the skin is closed, and a light compressive dressing is applied. Postoperative radiographs are obtained at the 6-week follow-up visit (**Fig. 7**).

POSTOPERATIVE MANAGEMENT

Immediate full weight bearing is permitted postoperatively in a stiff-soled shoe, and sutures are removed after 12 to 14 days. Physical therapy is initiated after suture removal and should focus on first MTP dorsiflexion and the resumption of a normal

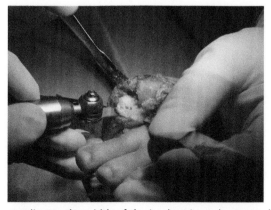

Fig. 4. A cut corresponding to the width of the implant is made perpendicular to the long axis of the proximal phalanx, making sure to preserve the sesamoid attachments.

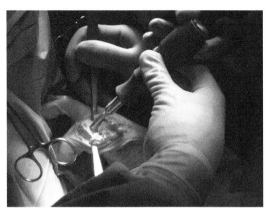

Fig. 5. Placement of keel punch into the proximal phalanx before implant insertion.

gait pattern. This rehabilitation program should continue for at least 4 months to prevent joint scarring and stiffness. Joint manipulation under anesthesia is considered if satisfactory motion is not obtained by 4 to 6 weeks after surgery.

DISCUSSION

Several studies have examined the clinical outcomes of first MTP hemiarthroplasty. Townley and Taranow[17] reported 95% good or excellent results in 279 implants with a maximum follow-up of 33 years using the BioPro (BioPro, Inc, Port Huron, MI, USA) first MTP joint hemiarthroplasty. A total of 13 of the 279 implants failed, with most failures occurring in patients with hallux valgus or rheumatoid arthritis. Most patients had encouraging long-term results, which supported the use of this technique in properly selected patients.

In a more recent study, Giza and colleagues[40] reviewed the results of 22 BioPro hemiarthroplasties performed on 20 patients. Visual analog scale (VAS) pain scores improved from 5 to 2.5 at 6 weeks during which time painless ambulation was generally observed. Range of motion improved 15° from an average of 32.7° preoperatively

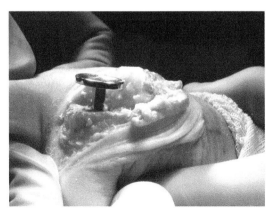

Fig. 6. Implant positioning in the proximal phalanx before final insertion with thumb pressure.

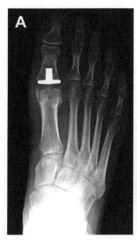
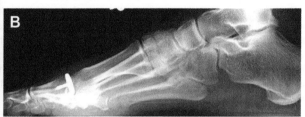

Fig. 7. Postoperative anteroposterior (A) and lateral (B) radiographs of the foot.

to 48.1° postoperatively, and the American Orthopaedic Foot and Ankle Society(AO-FAS) scores increased from 61 to 86 at 12 months. Complications included superficial wound infection, postoperative stiffness, and transfer metatarsalgia, with a complication rate of 18%.

Taranow and colleagues[44] reported improved Foot and Function Index scores and a high patient satisfaction rate after proximal phalangeal metallic hemiarthroplasty in patients with moderate to severe hallux rigidus. Sorbie and Saunders[6] also demonstrated favorable long-term results after hemiarthroplasty, with an increase in average AOFAS scores from 57 to 88 at a mean follow-up of 68 months. They found that the procedure alleviated stiffness and pain while preserving joint mobility, strength, and alignment.

Konkel and colleagues[45] published good to excellent results in 88% of patients during an average 6-year follow-up period using a Futura hemi-great toe implant. Both AOFAS and Koenig scores improved markedly, and a 76% increase in range of motion was documented. Of 23 patients, 19 were pain-free, whereas 4 patients experienced mild to moderate pain. Konkel and Menger[46] reviewed the midterm results of the Swanson titanium hemi-great toe prosthesis. Despite a high patient satisfaction rate of 85% at an average follow-up of 5.5 years, they noted prominent implant subsidence. In both studies, radiolucency was frequently observed around the implants despite the favorable outcomes.

Several studies have compared the available surgical treatments for hallux rigidus with mixed conclusions. Kim and colleagues[47] examined the results of arthrodesis, resectional arthroplasty, and hemi-implant and found no statistically significant difference in AOFAS or the American College of Foot and Ankle Surgeons scores at a mean postoperative follow-up of 159 weeks. Complications for the hemi-implant group included bony overgrowth, radiolucencies, and cystic change around the implant; dorsal drift of the hallux; and metatarsalgia. It was also noted that patients who underwent the hemi-implant procedure had a significantly lower average body mass index.

Raikin and colleagues[48] reported that only 57% of procedures using a metallic hemiarthroplasty had good or excellent results in comparison to 81% of arthrodesis procedures. The hemiarthroplasty group had a failure rate of 24%, with 5 failures requiring revision to address pain and aseptic loosening of the prosthesis. The mean postoperative AOFAS-HMI score at final follow-up was significantly higher for the arthrodesis group at 93.1% compared with 71.8% for the hemiarthroplasty group. The VAS pain score for the arthrodesis group was 1.7 points lower. The retrospective nature of this study may have influenced preoperative scoring.

Ghalambor and colleagues[49] analyzed histologic findings in 2 cases in which proximal phalanx titanium implants were removed and subsequent MTP arthrodesis was performed. They observed the presence of fibrous tissue and metallic debris located at the implant-bone interface. Mononuclear cells were also detected, which indicated osteolysis implant loosening in each of the cases.

Despite recent advancements and new techniques in implant arthroplasty, arthrodesis remains the treatment of choice for late-stage hallux rigidus.[16] Coughlin and Shurnas reported 100% good or excellent results in patients who underwent arthrodesis with a fusion rate of 94% (n = 34).[14] Goucher and Coughlin[50] found a fusion rate of 92% and patient satisfaction rate of 96%. Gibson and Thomson[51] reported similar results, with a significant improvement in pain scores after arthrodesis and no cases of nonunion.

Arthrodesis of the first MTP joint is a successful procedure, but pain is eliminated at the expense of joint mobility and function, which can have a significant impact on activity. This procedure can lead to changes in gait biomechanics and load distribution.[52] The proximal phalangeal hemiarthroplasty is a motion-preservation technique that also adequately addresses pain.[41] It is a uncomplicated procedure with a shortened recovery period and satisfactory results.

SUMMARY

Multiple treatment options exist for the management of late-stage hallux rigidus. The goals of treatment are pain reduction and restoration of function. Arthrodesis remains the treatment of choice, but recent advances support the use of first MTP hemiarthroplasty as a viable and successful option in properly selected patients in whom preservation of motion and function are desirable.

REFERENCES

1. Dellenbaugh SG, Bustillo J. Arthritides of the foot. Med Clin North Am 2014;98(2): 253–65.
2. Coughlin MJ, Shurnas PS. Hallux rigidus: demographics, etiology, and radiographic assessment. Foot Ankle Int 2003;24(10):731–43.
3. Iagnocco A, Rizzo C, Gattamelata A, et al. Osteoarthritis of the foot: a review of the current state of knowledge. Med Ultrason 2013;15(1):35–40.
4. Yee G, Lau J. Current concepts review: hallux rigidus. Foot Ankle Int 2008;29(6): 637–46.
5. Johnson JE, McCormick JJ. Modified oblique Keller capsular interposition arthroplasty (MOKCIA) for treatment of late-stage hallux rigidus. Foot Ankle Int 2014; 35(4):415–22.
6. Sorbie C, Saunders GA. Hemiarthroplasty in the treatment of hallux rigidus. Foot Ankle Int 2008;29(3):273–81.
7. Beeson P, Phillips C, Corr S, et al. Classification systems for hallux rigidus: a review of the literature. Foot Ankle Int 2008;29(4):407–14.
8. Polzer H, Polzer S, Brumann M, et al. Hallux rigidus: joint preserving alternatives to arthrodesis - a review of the literature. World J Orthop 2014;5(1):6–13.
9. Smith RW, Katchis SD, Ayson LC. Outcomes in hallux rigidus patients treated nonoperatively: a long-term follow-up study. Foot Ankle Int 2000;21(11):906–13.

10. DeCarbo WT, Lupica J, Hyer CF. Modern techniques in hallux rigidus surgery. Clin Podiatr Med Surg 2011;28(2):361–83, ix.
11. Hattrup SJ, Johnson KA. Subjective results of hallux rigidus following treatment with cheilectomy. Clin Orthop Relat Res 1988;(226):182–91.
12. Geldwert JJ, Rock GD, McGrath MP, et al. Cheilectomy: still a useful technique for grade I and grade II hallux limitus/rigidus. J Foot Surg 1992;31(2):154–9.
13. Mackay DC, Blyth M, Rymaszewski LA. The role of cheilectomy in the treatment of hallux rigidus. J Foot Ankle Surg 1997;36(5):337–40.
14. Coughlin MJ, Shurnas PS. Hallux rigidus. Grading and long-term results of operative treatment. J Bone Joint Surg Am 2003;85-A(11):2072–88.
15. Maffulli N, Papalia R, Palumbo A, et al. Quantitative review of operative management of hallux rigidus. Br Med Bull 2011;98:75–98.
16. Deland JT, Williams BR. Surgical management of hallux rigidus. J Am Acad Orthop Surg 2012;20(6):347–58.
17. Townley CO, Taranow WS. A metallic hemiarthroplasty resurfacing prosthesis for the hallux metatarsophalangeal joint. Foot Ankle Int 1994;15(11):575–80.
18. Johnson KA, Buck PG. Total replacement arthroplasty of the first metatarsophalangeal joint. Foot Ankle Int 1981;1(6):307–14.
19. Coutts A, Kilmartin TE, Ellis MJ. The long-term patient focused outcomes of the Keller's arthroplasty for the treatment of hallux rigidus. Foot (Edinb) 2012;22(3):167–71.
20. Coughlin MJ, Shurnas PJ. Soft-tissue arthroplasty for hallux rigidus. Foot Ankle Int 2003;24(9):661–72.
21. Coughlin MJ, Abdo RV. Arthrodesis of the first metatarsophalangeal joint with Vitallium plate fixation. Foot Ankle Int 1994;15(1):18–28.
22. Granberry WM, Noble PC, Bishop JO, et al. Use of a hinged silicone prosthesis for replacement arthroplasty of the first metatarsophalangeal joint. J Bone Joint Surg Am 1991;73(10):1453–9.
23. Hamilton WG, O'Malley MJ, Thompson FM, et al. Roger Mann Award 1995. Capsular interposition arthroplasty for severe hallux rigidus. Foot Ankle Int 1997;18(2):68–70.
24. Sanhudo JA, Gomes JE, Rodrigo MK. Surgical treatment of advanced hallux rigidus by interpositional arthroplasty. Foot Ankle Int 2011;32(4):400–6.
25. Merkle PF, Sculco TP. Prosthetic replacement of the first metatarsophalangeal joint. Foot Ankle Int 1989;9(6):267–71.
26. Coughlin MJ, Mann RA. Arthrodesis of the first metatarsophalangeal joint as salvage for the failed Keller procedure. J Bone Joint Surg Am 1987;69(1):68–75.
27. Flamme CH, Wulker N, Kuckerts K, et al. Follow-up results 17 years after resection arthroplasty of the great toe. Arch Orthop Trauma Surg 1998;117(8):457–60.
28. McNeil DS, Baumhauer JF, Glazebrook MA. Evidence-based analysis of the efficacy for operative treatment of hallux rigidus. Foot Ankle Int 2013;34(1):15–32.
29. Coughlin MJ. Arthrodesis of the first metatarsophalangeal joint with mini-fragment plate fixation. Orthopedics 1990;13(9):1037–44.
30. Erdil M, Elmadag NM, Polat G, et al. Comparison of arthrodesis, resurfacing hemiarthroplasty, and total joint replacement in the treatment of advanced hallux rigidus. J Foot Ankle Surg 2013;52(5):588–93.
31. Fitzgerald JA. A review of long-term results of arthrodesis of the first metatarsophalangeal joint. J Bone Joint Surg Br 1969;51(3):488–93.
32. Rajczy RM, McDonald PR, Shapiro HS, et al. First metatarsophalangeal joint arthrodesis. Clin Podiatr Med Surg 2012;29(1):41–9.
33. von Salis-Soglio G, Thomas W. Arthrodesis of the metatarsophalangeal joint of the great toe. Arch Orthop Trauma Surg 1979;95(1–2):7–12.

34. Dos Santos AL, Duarte FA, Seito CA, et al. Hallux rigidus: prospective study of joint replacement with hemiarthroplasty. Acta Ortop Bras 2013;21(2):71–5.
35. Shereff MJ, Jahss MH. Complications of silastic implant arthroplasty in the hallux. Foot Ankle Int 1980;1(2):95–101.
36. Fuhrmann RA, Wagner A, Anders JO. First metatarsophalangeal joint replacement: the method of choice for end-stage hallux rigidus? Foot Ankle Clin 2003; 8(4):711–21, vi.
37. Kitaoka HB, Holiday AD Jr, Chao EY, et al. Salvage of failed first metatarsophalangeal joint implant arthroplasty by implant removal and synovectomy: clinical and biomechanical evaluation. Foot Ankle Int 1992;13(5):243–50.
38. Mann RA. Surgical implications of biomechanics of the foot and ankle. Clin Orthop Relat Res 1980;(146):111–8.
39. Blair MP, Brown LA. Hallux limitus/rigidus deformity: a new great toe implant. J Foot Ankle Surg 1993;32(3):257–62.
40. Giza E, Sullivan M, Ocel D, et al. First metatarsophalangeal hemiarthroplasty for hallux rigidus. Int Orthop 2010;34(8):1193–8.
41. Perler AD, Nwosu V, Christie D, et al. End-stage osteoarthritis of the great toe/hallux rigidus: a review of the alternatives to arthrodesis: implant versus osteotomies and arthroplasty techniques. Clin Podiatr Med Surg 2013;30(3):351–95.
42. Ess P, Hamalainen M, Leppilahti J. Non-constrained titanium-polyethylene total endoprosthesis in the treatment of hallux rigidus. A prospective clinical 2-year follow-up study. Scand J Surg 2002;91(2):202–7.
43. Vanore JV, Christensen JC, Kravitz SR, et al. Diagnosis and treatment of first metatarsophalangeal joint disorders. Section 2: hallux rigidus. J Foot Ankle Surg 2003;42(3):124–36.
44. Taranow WS, Moutsatson MJ, Cooper JM. Contemporary approaches to stage II and III hallux rigidus: the role of metallic hemiarthroplasty of the proximal phalanx. Foot Ankle Clin 2005;10(4):713–28, ix–x.
45. Konkel KF, Menger AG, Retzlaff SA. Results of metallic hemi-great toe implant for grade III and early grade IV hallux rigidus. Foot Ankle Int 2009;30(7):653–60.
46. Konkel KF, Menger AG. Mid-term results of titanium hemi-great toe implants. Foot Ankle Int 2006;27(11):922–9.
47. Kim PJ, Hatch D, Didomenico LA, et al. A multicenter retrospective review of outcomes for arthrodesis, hemi-metallic joint implant, and resectional arthroplasty in the surgical treatment of end-stage hallux rigidus. J Foot Ankle Surg 2012;51(1): 50–6.
48. Raikin SM, Ahmad J, Pour AE, et al. Comparison of arthrodesis and metallic hemiarthroplasty of the hallux metatarsophalangeal joint. J Bone Joint Surg Am 2007; 89(9):1979–85.
49. Ghalambor N, Cho DR, Goldring SR, et al. Microscopic metallic wear and tissue response in failed titanium hallux metatarsophalangeal implants: two cases. Foot Ankle Int 2002;23(2):158–62.
50. Goucher NR, Coughlin MJ. Hallux metatarsophalangeal joint arthrodesis using dome-shaped reamers and dorsal plate fixation: a prospective study. Foot Ankle Int 2006;27(11):869–76.
51. Gibson JN, Thomson CE. Arthrodesis or total replacement arthroplasty for hallux rigidus: a randomized controlled trial. Foot Ankle Int 2005;26(9):680–90.
52. DeFrino PF, Brodsky JW, Pollo FE, et al. First metatarsophalangeal arthrodesis: a clinical, pedobarographic and gait analysis study. Foot Ankle Int 2002;23(6): 496–502.

Operative Technique

Interposition Arthroplasty and Biological Augmentation of Hallux Rigidus Surgery

Chad M. Ferguson, MD[a], J. Kent Ellington, MD, MS[b],*

KEYWORDS

- Interposition arthroplasty • Hallux rigidus • Surgical technique • Biologics • Amniox

KEY POINTS

- Interposition arthroplasty represents an effective alternative to joint arthroplasty for patients with grade 3 or 4 hallux rigidus.
- Grade C evidence supports the use of interposition arthroplasty for hallux rigidus.
- New techniques of biological augmentation propose unique solutions to perform interposition.

INTRODUCTION

Hallux rigidus is a common condition afflicting the first metatarsophalangeal (MTP) joint, caused by local degenerative changes, with resultant pain, synovitis, and restricted range of motion of the hallux MTP joint.[1-3] As the process advances, dorsal and dorsolateral osteophytes become evident clinically and radiographically (**Table 1**). This final common pathway may be the result of several individual pathologies including posttraumatic, inflammatory, and primary arthritides.[4] Many nonoperative modalities have been advocated for symptom control, including shoe modification, nonsteroidal antiinflammatory medication, local corticosteroid injection, and activity modification. Surgical care is recommended for cases refractory to conservative management. Many procedures have been described for treatment of this condition, which can be broadly characterized as joint preserving and joint sacrificing. Joint preservation options include cheilectomy, osteotomy, and combined cheilectomy with

J.K. Ellington is a stockholder, consultant, and teaching faculty for Amniox Medical. C.M. Ferguson has nothing to disclose.
[a] Department of Orthopaedic Surgery, Carolinas Medical Center, 1025 Morehead Medical Drive, Suite 300, Charlotte, NC 28204, USA; [b] OrthoCarolina, Foot and Ankle Institute, 2001 Vail Avenue #200b, Charlotte, NC 28207, USA
* Corresponding author.
E-mail address: Kentellingtonfx@gmail.com

Table 1
Clinical-radiographic system for grading hallux rigidus

Grade	Dorsiflexion	Radiographic Findings	Clinical Findings
0	40°–60° and/or 10%–20% loss compared with normal side	Normal	No pain; only stiffness and loss of motion on examination
1	30°–40° and/or 20%–50% loss compared with normal side	Dorsal osteophyte is main finding, minimal joint-space narrowing, minimal periarticular sclerosis, minimal flattening of metatarsal head	Mild or occasional pain and stiffness, pain at extremes of dorsiflexion and/or plantar flexion on examination
2	10°–30° and/or 50%–75% loss compared with normal side	Dorsal, lateral, and possibly medial osteophytes giving flattened appearance to metatarsal head, no more than one-quarter of dorsal joint space involved on lateral radiograph, mild to moderate joint-space narrowing and sclerosis, sesamoids not usually involved	Moderate to severe pain and stiffness, which may be constant; pain occurs just before maximum dorsiflexion and maximum plantar flexion on examination
3	≤10° and/or 75%–100% loss compared with normal side. There is notable loss of MTP plantar flexion as well (often ≤10° of plantar flexion)	Same as in grade 2 but with substantial narrowing, possibly periarticular cystic changes, more than one-quarter of dorsal joint space involved on lateral radiograph, sesamoids enlarged and/or cystic and/or irregular	Nearly constant pain and substantial stiffness at extremes of range of motion but not at midrange
4	Same as in grade 3	Same as in grade 3	Same criteria as grade 3 but there is definite pain at midrange of passive motion

Weight bearing and anteroposterior and lateral radiographs are used for radiographic assessment.
From Coughlin MJ, Shurnas PS. Hallux rigidus. Grading and long-term results of operative treatment. J Bone Joint Surg Am 2003;85-A(11):2073; with permission.

osteotomy. Joint sacrificing surgeries include arthrodesis, arthroplasty options with nontissue implant, resection arthroplasty, and interposition arthroplasty. Various levels of evidence are provided in the literature for these individual procedures (**Table 2**).[5]

Each of the surgical options offers unique advantages and disadvantages. Joint preservation surgery allows for preservation of motion, with improvement of pain in many patients; however, this operation does not address the fundamental degeneration, and therefore, pain recurrence is commonplace. Arthrodesis, contrarily, removes the motion and pain at the site of disease but causes alteration of gait[6] and is associated with complications such as malunion, nonunion, shortening, and transfer metatarsalgia.[7] Despite these shortcomings, most studies of outcomes for first MTP fusion have a high success rate.[8–10] With these considerations, hybrid procedures such as interposition arthroplasty and nonbiological implant arthroplasty can preserve

Table 2
Grades of recommendation for summaries or review of orthopedic surgical studies

Grade	Evidence
A	Good evidence (level I studies with consistent findings) for or against recommending intervention
B	Fair evidence (level II or III studies with consistent findings) for or against recommending intervention
C	Poor-quality evidence (level IV or V studies with consistent findings) for or against recommending intervention
I	There is insufficient or conflicting evidence not allowing a recommendation for against intervention

From Wright JG. Revised grades of recommendation for summaries or reviews of orthopaedic surgical studies. J Bone Joint Surg Am 2006;88(5):1161; with permission.

motion as well as address the disease process by removing portions of the degenerated joint and theoretically decrease the need for secondary procedures.[4]

Both joint preserving and joint sacrificing procedures have evidence for their efficacy to varying degrees. A recent review of the literature has made graded recommendations for each of these procedures and concluded that there is grade C evidence in support of cheilectomy, osteotomy, implant arthroplasty, resection arthroplasty, and interposition arthroplasty for treatment of hallux rigidus. In addition, the investigators concluded that grade B evidence exists in support of arthrodesis for hallux rigidus.[5]

Resection arthroplasty in isolation has been used successfully to treat hallux rigidus; however, in young, active patients, a flaccid and nonfunctional hallux can produce unsatisfactory outcomes.[3] For this reason, various types of interposition arthroplasty techniques have been described (**Table 3**).[3,4,11]

Indications for interposition arthroplasty include grade 3 and 4 hallux rigidus. Several studies have undertaken to compare interposition arthroplasty with other common joint salvage procedures. Lau and colleagues[12] showed no statistical difference in outcomes of patients treated with cheilectomy versus interposition arthroplasty in their retrospective cohort, with overall improvement in each group in American Orthopaedic Foot and Ankle Society (AOFAS), Short Form 36, and Visual Analog Scale (VAS) pain scores. Overall, both groups were satisfied with the result of the procedure.

Table 3
Indications for Keller resection arthroplasty

Indications	Contraindication
Indications	General Contraindications
• Failure of conservative treatment	• Medically unsuitable for surgery
• Stage 3–4 hallux rigidus	• Vascular insufficiency
• Lifestyle and shoe wear preferences that prevent arthrodesis	• Active infection, wound, or ulceration
• Age: fourth–eighth decade	• Neuropathy (relative)
	Specific Contraindications
	• Long second metatarsal (potential risk for development of transfer metatarsalgia)
	• Significant hallux valgus
	• Sesamoid arthritis
	• High-demand athletes
	• Inflammatory arthritis (relative)

Classically, interposition arthroplasty is conducted as a modified Keller resection arthroplasty combined with a dorsal capsular interposition to serve as a biological spacer.[3] Many investigators have suggested additional surgical modifications with alternative interpositions (**Table 3**).[13–15]

SURGICAL TECHNIQUE/PROCEDURE
Preoperative Planning

Office examination of the patient should be conducted, with examination of the affected foot. Comprehensive physical examination should be conducted, including inspection of skin condition, intact distal perfusion with palpable pulses, and presence of capillary refill, as well as focused examination of the hallux MTP joint showing presence of osteophytes, limitation of range of motion, and pain at extremes of range of motion. Comparison with the other foot is often helpful. Diagnosis is established with standard radiographic series, including weight bearing anteroposterior, oblique, and lateral radiographs showing joint-space narrowing of the hallux MTP joint and presence of a dorsal osteophyte with grading of stage 3 or stage 4 hallux rigidus. Physicians may consider use of a preoperative computed tomography scan for determination of the degree of MTP or sesamoid-metatarsal arthritis. If sesamoid arthritis is present, joint salvage procedure carries a high likelihood of failure, and hallux MTP fusion should be considered as an alternative.

Patient Positioning

The patient is positioned supine, with a bolster under the affected hip to rotate axis of the foot directed vertically on a radiolucent operative table. We prefer to use regional anesthesia with an ankle or popliteal block with intravenous sedation to minimize postoperative effects of general anesthesia. Preoperative intravenous prophylactic antibiotics are administered. In addition, a peripheral tourniquet is applied after exsanguination of the foot. A mini c-arm is placed on the ipsilateral side of the bed.

Surgical Approach

Our preferred technique: as initially described by Hamilton and colleagues,[11] a dorsal-medial longitudinal incision is made over the hallux MTP joint, with care to protect the dorsal and plantar medial cutaneous nerve. The incision should extend 2 cm distal and 4 cm proximal to the joint line. A dorsal incision over the extensor hallucis longus (EHL) tendon has been advocated by other investigators, because this facilitates exposure and access to the dorsomedial osteophyte with minimal retraction.[3]

Surgical Procedure

The following surgical technique describes the modified oblique Keller capsular interposition arthroplasty as initially described by Hamilton and colleagues[11]

1. The extensor hood is incised and the extensor hallucis brevis (EHB) and EHL tendons are separated and the EHB is transected and mobilized 3 cm proximal to the joint to prevent dynamic retraction during gait.
2. A longitudinal full-thickness midaxial capsulotomy is performed to expose the dorsal metatarsal and base of the proximal phalanx. The dorsal capsule and EHB are then elevated in a subperiosteal fashion from its insertion on the proximal phalanx with maximal length preservation (**Fig. 1**).
3. The dorsal structures are bluntly retracted laterally and a dorsal metatarsal cheilectomy is subsequently performed, removing the dorsal 25% to 33% of the

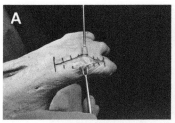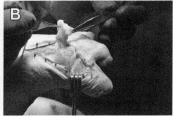

Fig. 1. Incision with longitudinal full-thickness midaxial capsulotomy of the dorsal hallux MTP joint with delineation of the dorsal capsular flap.

metatarsal head. Peripheral osteophytes should be removed, with special care to remove the dorsal-medial osteophyte (**Fig. 2**).

4. If required, a McGlamry elevator can be used to release the plantar base adhesions of the capsular reflection and the flexor hallucis brevis (FHB)/flexor hallucis longus (FHL) complex, with care to preserve these structures (**Fig. 3**).
5. Importantly, the metatarsal sesamoidal articulation should be visualized, because this may represent a postoperative pain generator, and understanding the condition of this joint can allow for guided patient expectations, or an alternative procedure (ie, arthrodesis) can be conducted (**Fig. 4**).
6. While protecting the EHL and FHL tendons, a dorsal oblique 8 mm metatarsal base osteotomy is performed with an oscillating saw, and the base of the proximal phalanx is removed. Care is taken during this step to avoid violation of the plantar attachment of the FHB and plantar plate at the base of the proximal phalanx, because iatrogenic injury can lead to a late cock-up deformity (**Fig. 5**).
7. A pin distractor is used to distract the base of the remaining phalanx and the metatarsal to allow for visualization of the dorsal and plantar structures.
8. The dorsal capsule-EHL complex is mobilized into the MTP joint dorsally and a nonabsorbable 2-0 suture is provisionally placed, anchoring it into the plantar plate/FHB complex plantarly. Provisional sutures should be placed laterally to medially and tied sequentially to avoid obscuring visualization and advance the tissue into the joint (**Fig. 6**).
9. Intraoperative fluoroscopy should be used to confirm that soft tissue balancing and alignment have been achieved to realign any preexisting deformity.
10. A medial capsular closure is conducted to using 2-0 absorbable suture.

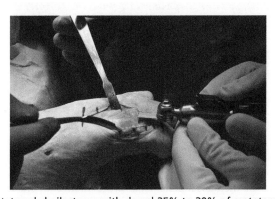

Fig. 2. Dorsal metatarsal cheilectomy with dorsal 25% to 30% of metatarsal head resected.

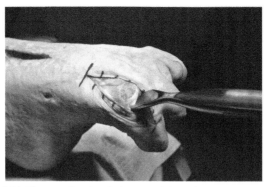

Fig. 3. Insertion of McGlamry elevator being used to gain exposure and elevate plantar capsule from plantar metatarsal head.

11. Skin is closed in standard fashion using the surgeon's preference.
12. Our preferred technique: a Kirschner wire is placed across the MTP joint to provide stability for the first 2 to 4 weeks postoperatively. This pin is removed during routine postoperative care (**Fig. 7**).

PUBLISHED MODIFICATIONS

Several investigators have suggested published modifications with alternative soft tissue interpositions, each with unique advantages, which are listed in the following sections.

Tendon Autograft Interposition

Coughlin and Shurnas[16] proposed the use of a free gracilis tendon autograft interposition. Other investigators have used other tendon donor grafts for similar techniques. As described by these investigators, the joint is approached as previously discussed. Subsequently, the proximal phalanx and distal metatarsal head are prepared with a cup-cone reamer system to a concave diameter of 14 to 16 mm. Using this technique, a spherical recess is formed. Subsequently, a 3-cm to 4-cm incision is made over the pes anserinus with dissection to the sartorial fascia. Fascial reflection exposes the

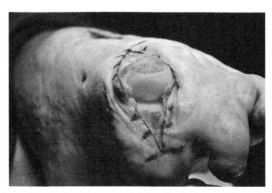

Fig. 4. Visualization of metatarsal sesamoidal articulation and evaluation of chondral articulations.

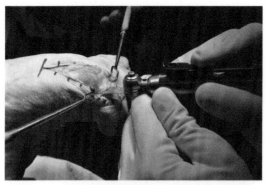

Fig. 5. Demonstration of a dorsal oblique 8 mm metatarsal base osteotomy. Care is taken to avoid violation of the plantar plate and FHB insertion.

underlying gracilis tendon, which is isolated using a tension suture distally and a tendon stripper to remove the tendon from its proximal origin. The tendon is prepared into a 15-mm sphere using a Ti-Cron suture and implanted in the MTP prepared cavity. Then, tendon interposition is sutured into the capsular closure to prevent migration. Closure is conducted as previously described (**Fig. 8**).

Regenerative Tissue Matrix

Berlet and colleagues[14,15] described a novel use of regenerative tissue matrix (GraftJacket matrix, Wright Medical Technology, Arlington, TN) for biological tissue implantation. As proposed for Coughlin and Shurnas[16] stage 3 hallux rigidus, this technique approaches the MTP joint as described in detail earlier. Bony preparation is undertaken by a thorough osteophyte removal and cheilectomy. When necessary, an additional modified Keller osteotomy can be performed to facilitate exposure. By the investigators' description, a rehydrated 5×5 cm^2 GraftJacket matrix (acellular allogenic dermal matrix), is fashioned circumferentially over the distal metatarsal head. An absorbable braded suture is used to secure the matrix through bone tunnels providing a biological resurfacing articulation (**Fig. 9**).

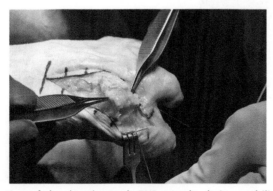

Fig. 6. Demonstration of the dorsal capsule-EHB complex being mobilized into the MTP joint dorsally. Sutures are used to affix the soft tissue flap plantarly into the FHB/plantar plate complex.

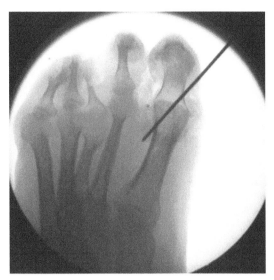

Fig. 7. Demonstration of a Kirschner wire being placed across the MTP joint to provide stability for the first 2 to 4 weeks postoperatively.

Fetal Amniotic Tissue Augmentation

Similar to the aforementioned biological matrix, Ellington and colleagues[17] have described the use of cryopreserved fetal amniotic membrane as a biological spacer and local antiinflammatory adjuvant. In this technique, the exposure is performed as outlined and a dorsal cheilectomy is performed. In contradistinction to conventional interposition arthroplasty, in this technique, a 2.5-cm² fetal cryopreserved amniotic tissue (Amniox, Amniox Medical, Atlanta, GA) is implanted over the cheilectomy bed; the tissue is not interposed between the hallux MTP articulation as with other discussed salvage options. The amniotic tissue is secured in place and routine closure follows. This technique relies on the decompression provided by the cheilectomy to allow for increased postoperative joint motion. Amniotic tissue has been shown to have a unique

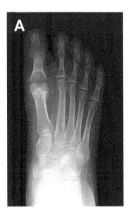
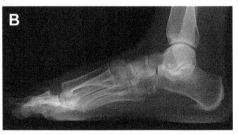

Fig. 8. Anteroposterior and lateral radiographs show postoperative images of a right foot with stage 3 hallux rigidus. The patient was treated with tendon autograft interposition as described. (*Courtesy of* Mark Myerson, MD, Baltimore, MD.)

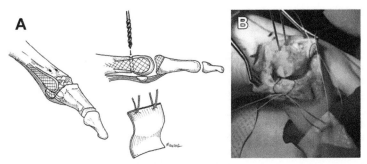

Fig. 9. (*A*) Regenerative tissue matrix technique and (*B*) intraoperative photograph. (*Courtesy of* Gregory C. Berlet, MD, Columbus, OH.)

biological function facilitating immunomodulation[18], preventing adhesions[19] and minimizing postoperative inflammation.[20] Hypothetically, this tissue mitigates the production of scar tissue and preserves postoperative range of motion. The usefulness of this tissue is under investigation by a prospective study (OrthoCarolina, Charlotte, NC). By extrapolating to the hallux rigidus in joint preserving and joint sacrificing procedures such as cheilectomy and interposition arthroplasty, the investigators seek to mitigate the adverse effects of postoperative scar tissue formation and stiffness in hallux MTP surgery (**Fig. 10**).

POSTOPERATIVE DRESSING
Dressing

Destabilization of the MTP joint during this procedure requires emphasis on the postoperative dressing to facilitate postoperative alignment. At the conclusion of the surgery, a sterile dressing is applied with nonadherent gauze over the incision site. A dressing of surgeon preference is applied. Importantly, the surgeon should ensure neutral alignment in the sagittal and coronal plan, which must be maintained in the postoperative period until healing has occurred (**Table 4**).[3,4,21]

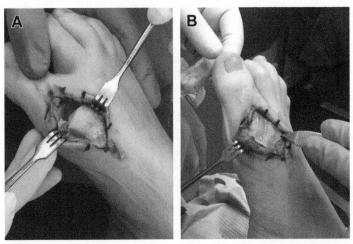

Fig. 10. Intraoperative photographs of fetal amniotic membrane implantation. (*A*) The cheilectomy bed decompressed and prepared for implantation. (*B*) The graft in place before soft tissue closure.

Table 4
Complications and management

Complication	Management
Infection, wound dehiscence, postoperative scar formation, and so forth	General complications of foot and ankle surgery are managed specific to the cause as based on surgeon experience
Specific Complications	
Dorsal and plantar medial cutaneous neurapraxia	Meticulous surgical technique can minimize the incidence. Symptomatic treatment includes systemic or local antineuropathic medication (ie, gabapentin), manual massage and desensitization, topical analgesics
Metatarsalgia	Postoperative metatarsalgia should be treated with accommodative shoe modification with metatarsal pad insertion
Cock-up toe	Complication can represent postoperative sequelae of inadvertent surgical release of the distal FHB from the proximal phalangeal attachment. Symptomatic treatment or arthrodesis is recommended

POSTOPERATIVE CARE

The postoperative modified oblique Keller interposition arthroplasty protocol is outlined in. No formal physical therapy is typically recommended in this protocol (**Fig. 11**).

OUTCOMES

Lau and colleagues[12] reported a retrospective cohort study of interposition arthroplasty (n = 11) compared with cheilectomy with dorsal closing wedge osteotomy (n = 24). In this study, patients with grade 2 hallux rigidus were treated with

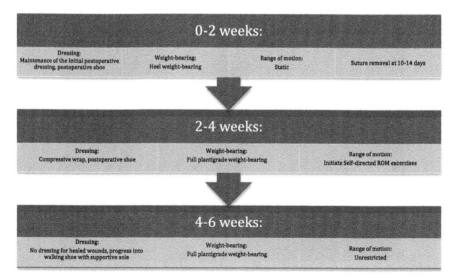

Fig. 11. Postoperative protocol represents our preferred protocol and may be modified if concomitant procedures are performed.

cheilectomy and grade 3 hallux rigidus with interposition arthroplasty. At average 24-month follow-up, no difference in AOFAS, Foot Function Index, or VAS pain scores, with good/excellent results in 8/11 and 21/24, respectively.

Mackey and colleagues[7] reported the results of their retrospective case series of patients selected to have modified oblique Keller capsular interposition arthroplasty (n = 10) to an arthrodesis group (n = 12). At mean 63-month follow-up, the interposition arthroplasty group reported higher AOFAS scores (AOFAS = 89.55) compared with arthrodesis (AOFAS = 64.48). In addition, the investigators showed significantly higher pressures under the great toe in the arthrodesis group.

Schenk and colleagues[22] reviewed a series of patients comparing Keller resection arthroplasty (n = 30) with modified oblique Keller capsular interposition arthroplasty (n = 22). Although the investigators were not able to show an improvement in the interposition arthroplasty group, both groups were found to have improvement in their AOFAS scores at 15-month follow-up. Keiserman and colleagues[23] have also shown overall improvement in a retrospective cohort.

OUTCOMES OF MODIFIED TECHNIQUES

Data are limited regarding modifications to the classic interposition arthroplasty. Autograft tendon as well as orthobiological augmentation have been advocated as a surgical modification for the dorsal capsule interposition as outlined. Overall, the results of these techniques have been reported by several studies to be comparable with classic interposition arthroplasty in functional patient outcomes.[3,15,16] Hyer and colleagues[15] reported am improvement from 38 to 65.8 at an average 5.4-year follow-up in a retrospective case series of 9 patients with regenerative tissue matrix interposition arthroplasty. In this patient cohort, no patient underwent revision surgery within the study period. Cryopreserved amniotic tissue is under study for usefulness in hallux rigidus treated with dorsal cheilectomy; however, no data are available regarding use for interposition arthroplasty.

SUMMARY

The objective in the treatment of hallux rigidus is to alleviate pain, maintain medial column plantar flexion strength, and restore or maintain function.[1] Interposition arthroplasty offers a motion-preserving alternative to arthrodesis, with grade C evidence to support its usefulness in hallux rigidus. Several modifications to the original procedures have been made, and several biological augmentations offer new procedures. Careful patient selection with appropriate expectations can yield excellent outcomes with this procedure. Larger prospective series with long-term follow-up are required to compare the results of these new procedures with their historical counterparts.

REFERENCES

1. Mann RA, Clanton TO. Hallux rigidus: treatment by cheilectomy. J Bone Joint Surg Am 1988;70(3):400–6.
2. Camasta CA. Hallux limitus and hallux rigidus. Clinical examination, radiographic findings, and natural history. Clin Podiatr Med Surg 1996;13(3):423–48.
3. Coughlin, Michael J. Mann's Surgery of the Foot and Ankle. 9th ed. Philadelphia: Saunders/Elsevier; 2014, in print.
4. Wiesel, Sam W. Operative Techniques in Orthopaedic Surgery. Philadelphia: Lippincott Williams & Wilkins; 2011, in print.

5. McNeil DS, Baumhauer JF. Evidence-based analysis of the efficacy for operative treatment of hallux rigidus. Foot Ankle Int 2013;34(1):15–32.
6. Brodsky JW, Baum BS, Pollo FE. Prospective gait analysis in patients with first metatarsophalangeal joint arthrodesis for hallux rigidus. Foot Ankle 2007;28(2):162–5.
7. Mackey RB. The modified oblique Keller capsular interpositional arthroplasty for hallux rigidus. J Bone Joint Surg Am 2010;92(10):1938.
8. Doty J, Coughlin M, Hirose C, et al. Hallux metatarsophalangeal joint arthrodesis with a hybrid locking plate and a plantar neutralization screw: a prospective study. Foot Ankle Int 2013;34(11):1535–40.
9. Beertema W, Draijer WF, van Os JJ, et al. A retrospective analysis of surgical treatment in patients with symptomatic hallux rigidus: long-term follow-up. J Foot Ankle Surg 2006;45(4):244–51.
10. Gibson J, Thomson CE. Arthrodesis or total replacement arthroplasty for hallux rigidus: a randomized controlled trial. Foot Ankle Int 2005;26(9):680–90.
11. Hamilton WG, O'Malley MJ, Thompson FM, et al. Roger Mann Award 1995. Capsular interposition arthroplasty for severe hallux rigidus. Foot Ankle Int 1997;18(2):68–70.
12. Lau J, Daniels TR. Outcomes following cheilectomy and interpositional arthroplasty in hallux rigidus. Foot Ankle Int 2001;22(6):462–70.
13. Coughlin MJ, Shurnas PS. Hallux rigidus. J Bone Joint Surg Am 2004;86-A(Suppl 1(Pt 2)):119–30.
14. Berlet GC, Hyer CF, Lee TH, et al. Interpositional arthroplasty of the first MTP joint using a regenerative tissue matrix for the treatment of advanced hallux rigidus. Foot Ankle Int 2008;29(1):10–21.
15. Hyer CF, Granata JD, Berlet GC, et al. Interpositional arthroplasty of the first metatarsophalangeal joint using a regenerative tissue matrix for the treatment of advanced hallux rigidus: 5-year case series follow-up. Foot Ankle Spec 2012; 5(4):249–52.
16. Coughlin MJ, Shurnas PJ. Soft-tissue arthroplasty for hallux rigidus. Foot Ankle Int 2003;24(9):661–72.
17. Ellington JK, Ferguson CM. The use of amniotic membrane/umbilical cord in first metatarsophalangeal joint cheilectomy: a comparative bilateral case study. Surg Technol Int 2014;25:63–7.
18. Liu J, Sheha H, Fu Y, et al. Update on amniotic membrane transplantation. Expert Rev Ophthalmol 2010;5(5):645–61.
19. Ozgenel GY. The effects of a combination of hyaluronic and amniotic membrane on the formation of peritendinous adhesions after flexor tendon surgery in chickens. J Bone Joint Surg Br 2004;86(2):301–7.
20. Shimmura S, Shimazaki J, Ohashi Y, et al. Antiinflammatory effects of amniotic membrane transplantation in ocular surface disorders. Cornea 2001;20(4): 408–13.
21. Johnson JE, McCormick JJ. Modified oblique Keller capsular interposition arthroplasty (MOKCIA) for treatment of late-stage hallux rigidus. Foot Ankle Int 2014; 35(4):415–22.
22. Schenk S, Meizer R, Kramer R, et al. Resection arthroplasty with and without capsular interposition for treatment of severe hallux rigidus. Int Orthop 2007; 33(1):145–50.
23. Keiserman LS, Sammarco VJ, Sammarco GJ. Surgical treatment of the hallux rigidus. Foot Ankle Clin 2005;10(1):75–96.

Index

Note: Page numbers of article titles are in **boldface** type.

Foot Ankle Clin N Am 20 (2015) 525–545
http://dx.doi.org/10.1016/S1083-7515(15)00070-4
1083-7515/15/$ – see front matter © 2015 Elsevier Inc. All rights reserved.

foot.theclinics.com

Moving?

Make sure your subscription moves with you!

To notify us of your new address, find your **Clinics Account Number** (located on your mailing label above your name), and contact customer service at:

Email: journalscustomerservice-usa@elsevier.com

800-654-2452 (subscribers in the U.S. & Canada)
314-447-8871 (subscribers outside of the U.S. & Canada)

Fax number: 314-447-8029

Elsevier Health Sciences Division
Subscription Customer Service
3251 Riverport Lane
Maryland Heights, MO 63043

*To ensure uninterrupted delivery of your subscription, please notify us at least 4 weeks in advance of move.

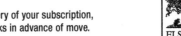

Printed and bound by CPI Group (UK) Ltd, Croydon, CR0 4YY

03/10/2024

01040492-0015